The Bariatric Keto ReStart Program

The 14 day Keto ReStart Program to help you start again and maximize your weight loss potential.

Mary Beth Filer

BARIATRIC KETO

Dedicated to the following :

To My Doctors:
One for saving my life (William A. Fintel, Oncology); one for helping me find my life's purpose (Mark D. Schueler, Chiropractor); one for giving me back a life worth living (Tananchai A. Lucktong, Bariatric Surgeon).
You will never know the tens of thousands of lives you have touched in a deeply positive way.

My eldest son, DJ, who shocked me out of complacency with his fear I would not live long enough to see grandchildren.

My husband, David, who has loved me at every size. ❤️

And most of all, to the administrators & moderators of Bariatric Keto who have seen me through dark days to the light of victory and GOAL WEIGHT! 🤣

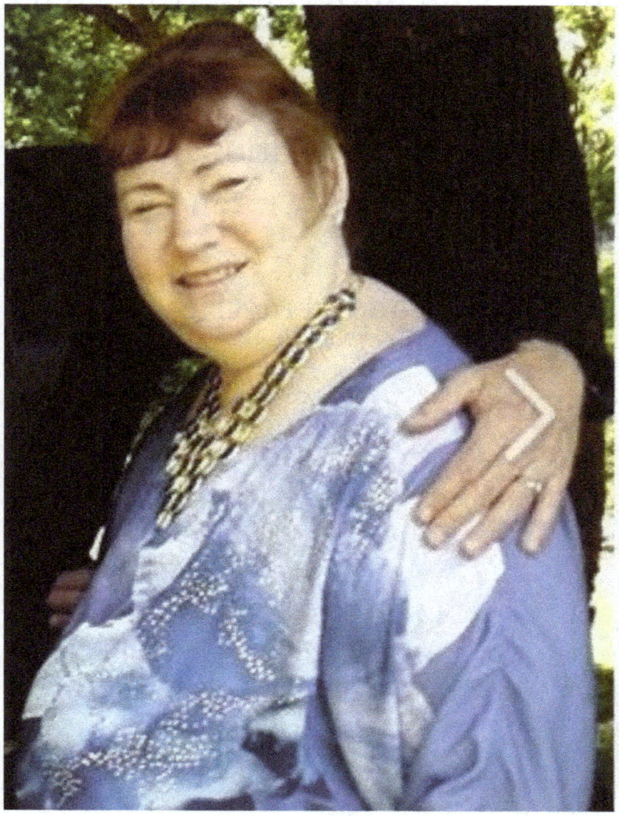

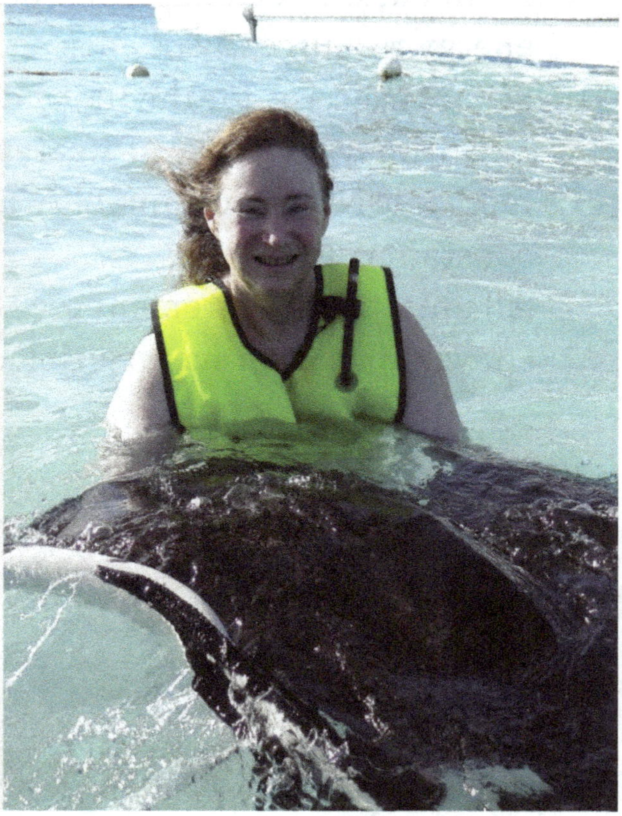

IMPORTANT INFORMATION

Content provided in this book is of a general nature only and does not replace the information and advice provided by your own health care team. Bariatric Keto and its affiliate programs are not recommended for those who have type 1 diabetes, heart disease, kidney disease, or any other disease state that requires continuous medical supervision. We do not endorse the cessation of any prescribed medications. Always consult your own health care providers for specific personal health and medical advice or to see if a program is right for you.

- ReStart should not be undertaken by anyone less than three months post-op.
- There should be a **minimum of 30 days (preferably 45 days)** from the end of one ReStart to the beginning of a new ReStart.
- Do not attempt a ReStart if you are ill. Wait until you have all your energy resources available.
- Do not exercise for the first **7 days** while on ReStart.
- The primary purpose of ReStart is to reset your relationship with food. It is NOT a sustainable way of eating. It is not intended for constant use.
- All units of measurement are U.S. We have added metric conversions wherever possible.

TABLE OF CONTENTS

Content provided in this book is of a general nature only and does not replace the information and advice provided by your own health care professionals. Always consult your own health care providers for specific personal health and medical advice.

I

The Process

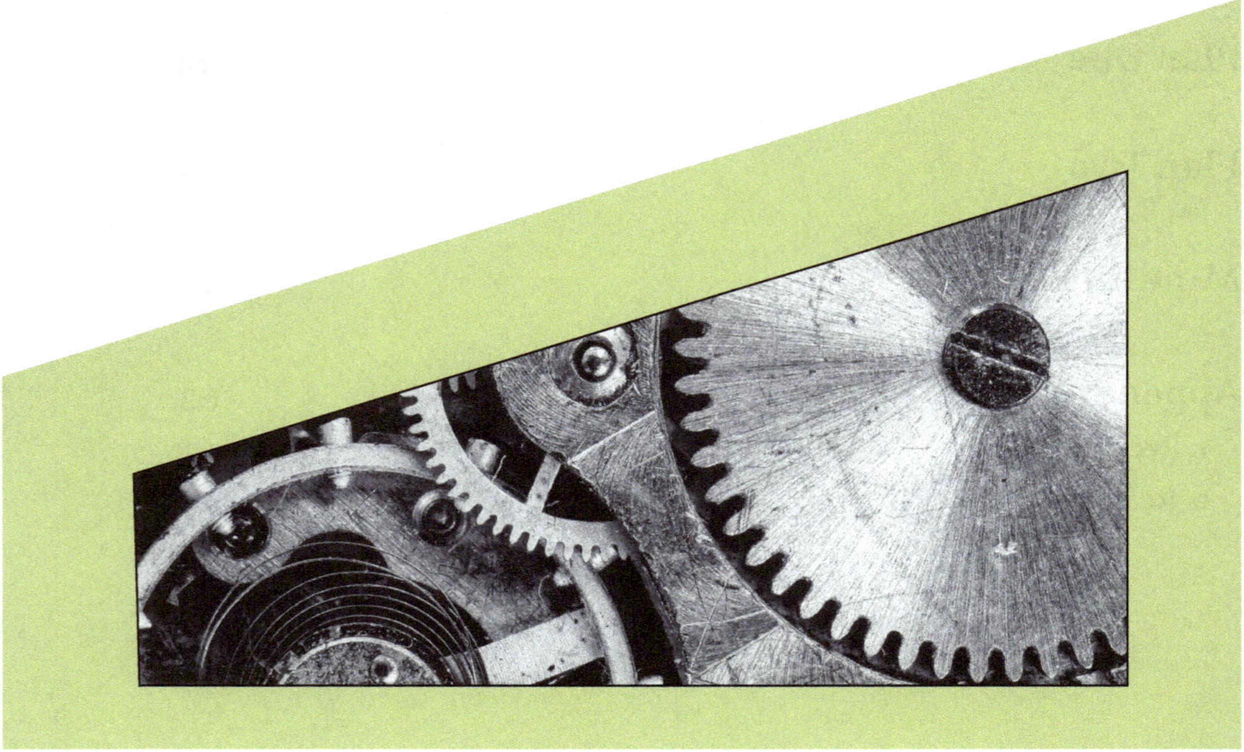

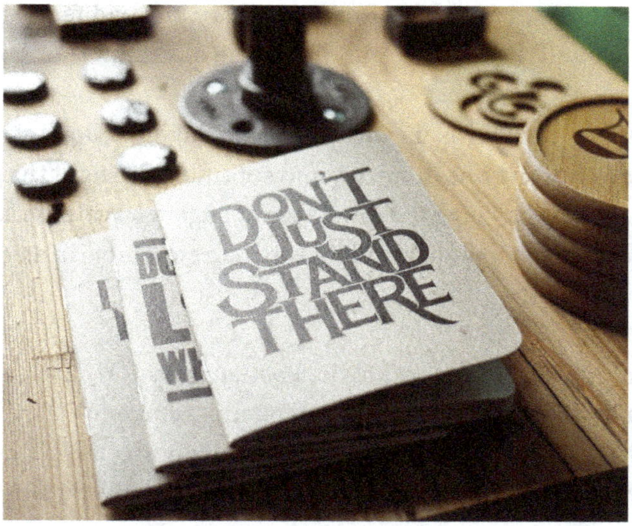

Ready to ReStart? Then STOP. Right NOW. Purchase a small container of Bragg's Apple Cider Vinegar (ACV) and try a shot in water. Hot or cold, you need to add water for your teeth & throat's sake. If it makes you squirm like you have a spider on you, then you need to order ACV capsules. Some people like ACV so much they add shots of tabasco and pepper. Others, like me, swear it could raise the dead and simply can't stomach the shots. That's why capsules were invented.

Next, look over the Shopping List. See what you already have and figure out a plan to get the rest. You can't start until you have everything in.

Everything ordered? Then take a deep breath and settle in for a short read....
Successful weight loss post WLS is a mind game. It's all in your head – not your stomach. I've often remarked I wish I had surgery on my brain rather than my stomach. The need to consume is driven by our heads rather than our bodies.

Food functioned as our best friend for many years prior to weight loss surgery. Where we laughed with friends over a sports game and celebrated holidays with family. Happy Birthday sung over a cake with candles, breakfast in bed for Mother's or Father's Day, s'mores by the campfire. Food has been an integral part of our lives since our first memories.

But food has also been our hidden shame. It is where we took refuge when the world was cruel. Eating our feelings was real for us. Many of us have come to look back and realize we were/are addicts. Addicted to the smells and textures and tastes that brought us so much happiness in the past. We consistently tried to recreate – and eat – our happy times whenever we could. But there was a problem. Although the plate in front of us was empty, the bad feelings didn't go away. They were always waiting just around the corner. And the shame of yet another failure stayed with us.

The food industry continually bombards us with messages saying, "Don't you deserve a treat today?" And, really, we do. Just for waking up one more day and continuing to fight the good fight – for ourselves, our families, our children. However – big food's message of sugary sweetness is making us fat. It's killing us. So much so that we allowed ourselves to be filleted on a surgical table in an effort to start again; to lose the excess weight and regain health.

Our relationship with food prior to surgery was toxic. Post-surgery, it HAS to change. We need to shed the old abusive relationship and look at food as simply an energy source--WITHOUT emotion. That doesn't mean it can't taste good. I never let anything pass my lips that doesn't make my tongue dance. Instead of quantity – go for high flavor impact and quality. Put your health and well being ahead of the urge to feed.

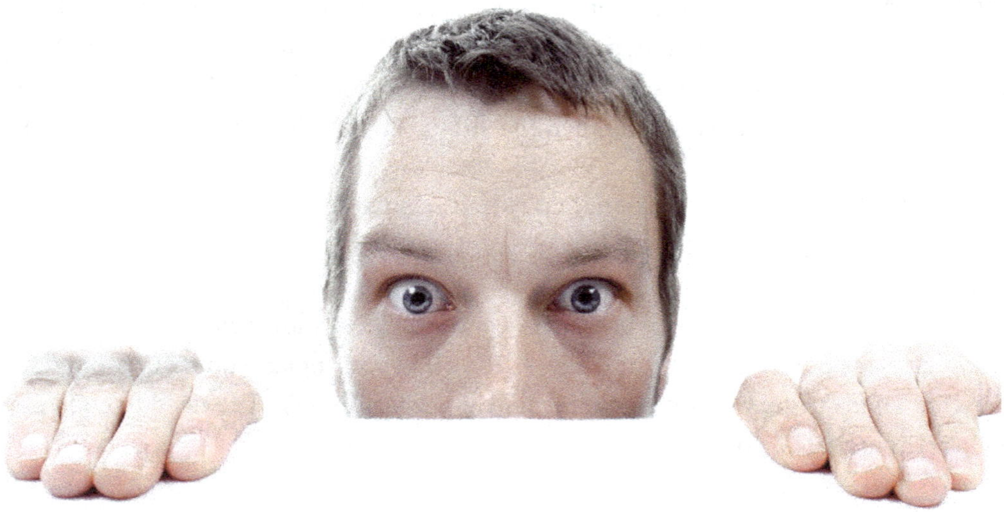

YOU SAY YOU'RE NERVOUS?

You would be shocked how many people tell me they're scared to begin ReStart. Is it fear of failure? Fear of change? Or maybe even fear of success?

Many of us have worked YEARS to get to where we are now, even if it's not where we want to eventually be. You've made it through the hard part - the decision to have weight loss surgery. You endured the anxiety before the surgery and the healing after. ReStart is a cake walk compared to where you've already

Content provided in this book is of a general nature only and does not replace the information and advice provided by your own health care professionals. Always consult your own health care providers for specific personal health and medical advice.

been. There is nothing to fear and health to gain. You can't fail on the program. You will ALWAYS learn something about yourself and your new body. You can start or stop whenever you like and use this tool again and again.

We do encourage you to complete the entire 14 day program for maximum results. Honestly, only the first 2 - 3 days are difficult. Personally, I could live with the devil for 2-3 days if it put goal weight within reach!

After those 2-3 tough days it's all downhill and results. So, no matter what else happens in your life, resolve to continue the program for at least 3 days. That's your success criteria. Every additional day on the program will bring greater insight, learning and weight loss.

Notice I listed weight loss last in that list. Until you get ALL of you - MIND & BODY - working on the same battle plan, you cannot hope to get to and maintain goal weight and a healthy life. It simply isn't possible. You have to want this change enough to bring it into existence. The mind work is every bit as important as the food work.

So grab a calendar and chart out your 14 days. Some prefer to start on a Monday and spend the rough time at work. I prefer to have Day 1 on a Friday. I don't get hangry until the evening of Day 1. So I take something to help me sleep and go to bed early. Honestly, I wouldn't subject ANYONE to being around me during DAYS 2 & 3. I send the family away for the weekend and have my own pity party. During it, I log into our Facebook ReStart group and console myself others are just as miserable - yet they make it through. That picture in my mind of me at goal weight in my goal weight dress gets me through the long days. Going to bed early and sleeping as long as possible keeps the late night carb munchies from crawling out from under the bed and attacking. By the end of the weekend my clothes fit better, I'm well rested and so proud of simply surviving. The family arrives back safe and sound, never knowing how close they came to hangry danger.

You say you're always hungry? I'll show you a program where you can tell the difference between real hunger and head hunger. Where you can get the scales moving back in the RIGHT direction. With a program that is only 14 days long – and really, what is 14 days compared to what you've already been

You can't start the next chapter of your
life if you keep rereading the last one.
-Unknown

through? Within those 14 days you'll know if Bariatric Keto is right for you. I promise you – I won't be insulted if it's not! No one program is right for everyone. The proof is in how you feel, how your clothes fit, and maybe in that little number on the scale.

AM I STRONG ENOUGH TO DO THIS?

You can only achieve what you believe you can achieve. Don't ALLOW ReStart to become another title on the list of failures. We'll show you coping strategies to get through a meeting without eating that donut. How to get past late-night carb munchies and remember the person you dreamed you could be when you first had WLS. Don't be willing to settle for less!

NO WORKOUTS ALLOWED!

During the first week of ReStart you're heavily restricting food intake. You may feel faint, weak or experience dizziness. This happens most with members who have undiagnosed thyroid issues, but can happen to anyone. Be gentle with your body the first week. Science has consistently shown us weight loss is 80% food restriction and 20% exercise. Unless you're an olympic athlete, taking a week off from the gym isn't going to impact your performance much. The risk from a fall outweighs any workout benefit.

Historically, the gym has been a place of punishment for obese people. Sure, there are exceptions, but most of us have practically killed ourselves on those machines trying to lose a few pounds, only to end up hurt. Your center of gravity is changing with your weight. With poor muscle strength comes poor recovery ability and coordination. We actually advise not hitting the gym until closer to goal weight.

But there are ways we can still enjoy getting our muscles flexing and blood pumping! Resistance bands, walking, yoga, simple stretching, flowing repetitive motion routines like QiGong or Y-Dan are encouraged starting the second week of ReStart. They will help you feel better, eliminate fluid retention and keep the weight coming off. Get in the habit of moving your body NOW - during the second week of ReStart. It will help you maintain the habit after ReStart.

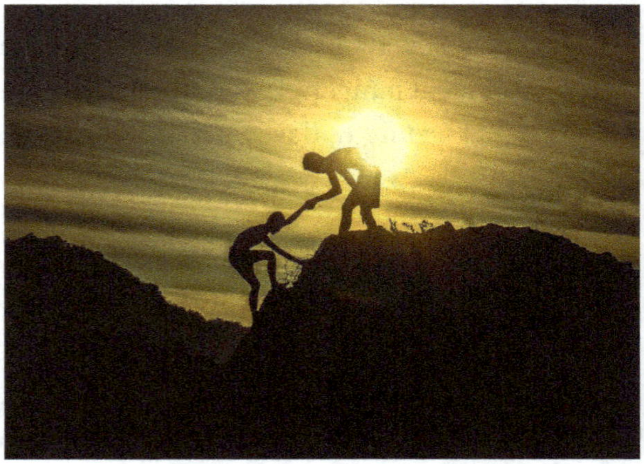

YOU'RE NOT IN THIS ALONE

There's no reason to try to walk the path to goal weight alone. You have MANY others walking

Content provided in this book is of a general nature only and does not replace the information and advice provided by your own health care professionals. Always consult your own health care providers for specific personal health and medical advice.

the same path. Why not give and take inspiration? We have dedicated support groups where you can discuss recipes, menus and everything else you can think of. Discover what makes others journey's easier and incorporate it into your own.

You need a support network. This fight is too big to handle on your own. It doesn't matter if the support comes from friends, family or fellow travelers on our groups. Eventually, we all need to lean on someone. Make sure that someone is well informed and wants only the best for you.

Your body reacts to carbs by packing on the pounds. As you unpack those pounds the hormones stored in them gets re-released into your bloodstream. Remember right after surgery the roller coaster of emotions you felt? That was courtesy of the hormones stored in your fat. As the fat is used for fuel, the hormones are re-released into the bloodstream. Those hormones cause you to feel the same emotions you felt while you were putting the fat on. Notice no one is cheering here. It's ugly, but a fact of weight gain is that traumatic events often trigger eating & weight gain. So chances are you're going to be experiencing some bad emotions while losing quickly. Tell your family to buckle their seat belts and hang on for the ride. The first week of ReStart can be kind of bumpy. I send my family away for a week of camping. It's FAR easier than having to spend the next month apologizing.

Our Facebook groups are:

Bariatric Keto for Women: https://www.facebook.com/groups/423596911345242

Bariatric Keto for Men: https://www.facebook.com/groups/117602878912804/

Bariatric Keto New Beginnings Pre-Surgery – 8 weeks: https://www.facebook.com/groups/168695337017658/

Bariatric Keto ReStart: https://www.facebook.com/groups/475119699553643/

Bariatric Keto Exercise: https://www.facebook.com/groups/2068319956783709/

Be Prepared

ALWAYS REMEMBER TO PLAN AHEAD

Your number one key to weight loss is planning ahead. As the Boy Scouts say, "Be Prepared". Keep a packet of Ultima along with some stevia in your purse/briefcase. Beef jerky or cheese crisps in your car, along with a few bottles of water. Caught out late? No problem. That's why you have emergency supplies prepared.

Live in a town where it's hard to get some ingredients? Order them now. You'll find a shopping list in Appendix C. Now is NOT the time to skimp on ingredient quality or you'll regret it later.
Select one day every weekend to precook most of your meals for the week. That way there's never a reason to have to grab lunch or dinner out.

Second, log everything that passes your lips. And I mean EVERYTHING. Weigh every portion using a food scale. When you eat to our menu plan your meals will be logged for you. But you'll still need to check off supplements & water consumption. EXCEPT on ReStart. Yes, I know – I just contradicted myself. The beauty of ReStart is there is NO counting. No macros to follow. You simply eat what's written on the page and watch the results roll in. BUT you can't stay on ReStart forever. It isn't a fully balanced eating program. In fact, we only recommend going through it no more than once every 3 months. It needs to be in your tool kit when the BIG GUNS are needed. You'll be shown other tools to use in your daily eating when you're trained in BariKeto.

Third, draw on support from your network. Don't forget to add your medical team in this circle. This will enable you to make more informed choices about food. You're welcome to share our resources with your medical team provided they are not copied and/or distributed. These are copyrighted works and must be purchased from us. If we all band together on this road to goal weight, no one will fail!

Fourth, mindfulness. It's a big word that simply means being aware in this moment. Not thinking about the past or future. Only NOW exists. By being present in the moment, we can achieve greater pleasure from the food we consume; become aware of our body's own full signal and not take "just one or two more bites"; learn to recognize and put a name to our feelings. We begin to recognize our feelings for what they are – and what they are not. Is your urge to consume stemming from:
A past memory of good times spent over food?
Smelling or seeing a food you used to love?
A disappointing interaction with someone?

"Mindful practices enhance the connection between our body, our mind and everything else that is around us. Mindful living is the key to understanding our struggles with weight and to empower us to control our weight."
~Thich Nhat Hanh

Mindfulness helps you put coping mechanisms in place to identify and then deal with emotions appropriately. The goal is to acknowledge the feeling, observe your body's response to the feeling, then let the feeling go. You cannot control everything that happens to you in life. But you CAN control how you respond to those things. Take back your power. Respond with observation rather than taking action.

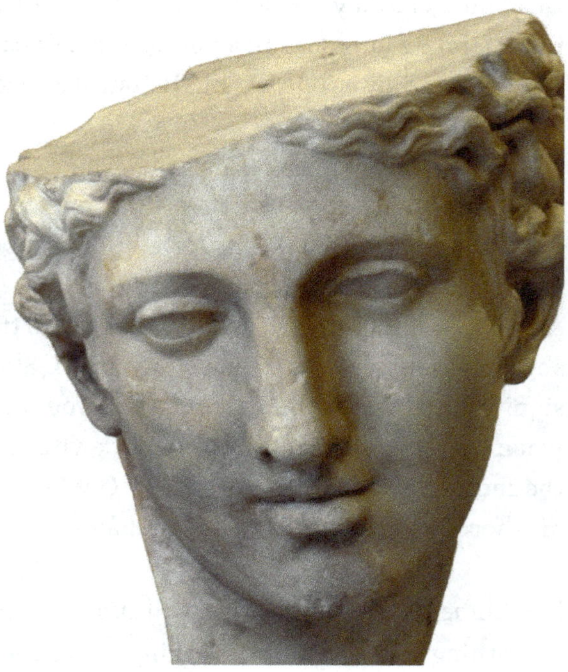

How do you do this? By being self-aware. Grant yourself the grace to take a few moments to pause and identify the feelings evoked by the message coming at you. What was the message and who did it come from? Observe your body's impulse to take action and what that action is. Then decide how you choose to respond.

I've shown you how to identify emotions that often lead to overeating. Next, you'll learn how to develop coping mechanisms to deal with those feelings constructively.

Content provided in this book is of a general nature only and does not replace the information and advice provided by your own health care professionals. Always consult your own health care providers for specific personal health and medical advice.

Coping Tools

Remember – observe the feeling without judgment. Look inward to discover the manifestation of the feeling. Do you feel cold; hungry; lonely? By putting a name to the feeling, you can cope with the feeling.

Bored? Go for a walk. Listen to music & dance. Sing at the top of your lungs. Order supplies.
Tired? Instead of a nap, pamper yourself. Paint your nails, try on clothes from your closet or drawers (we ALL have many sizes of clothing).

Head hunger? Play "What Will I Look Like After Plastics?" in the bathroom mirror. Get a massage.
Upset? Take a long soak in a hot Epsom Salt bath. Read a book. Meditate/pray to restore calm.
Depressed? Buy a GOAL WEIGHT outfit and look at it often, imagining yourself in it. Look at your progress photos.

Don't forget your support network! Login to the group and show someone the love & support you want to be shown. Be willing to accept the support offered and absorb the knowledge it provides.

ALWAYS, remove items/foods you know will trigger you. Significant other brought in food when he/she knew you were trying hard to avoid it? Stomp on the food. Then throw it in the garbage. Your significant other should be supporting your efforts, not sabotaging them. Always crave salty snacks when watching TV? Replace the snack with chips you can have, or better yet, don't sit down to watch the show. Stand & shuffle your feet. Get PMS and crave chocolate every month? Order 10 gram bars of ChocoPerfection to have on hand for these times.

Remember – denying yourself will simply lead to binging later. But the person who says, "Eat everything in moderation" is asking for a surgery revision. If we COULD have eaten everything in moderation, we WOULD have. Instead – learn what you can eat that's tasty and satisfying and makes your tongue dance. Quality instead of quantity. Because soon I'll show you that hunger you're feeling is likely all in your head.

Being mindful ensures you will succeed in your weight loss efforts. Allow yourself the grace to be human – with all the flaws that go along with it. By acknowledging the imperfection, you now have the opportunity to CHANGE it. No one ever changed anything because life was too damn good. We change only when we no longer are willing to accept the present.

NO ONE CHANGES VOLUNTARILY. CHANGE IS ALWAYS HARD. THE ONLY TIME CHANGE WILL HAPPEN IS WHEN YOU DECIDE THE CONSEQUENCES OF NOT CHANGING ARE HARDER.

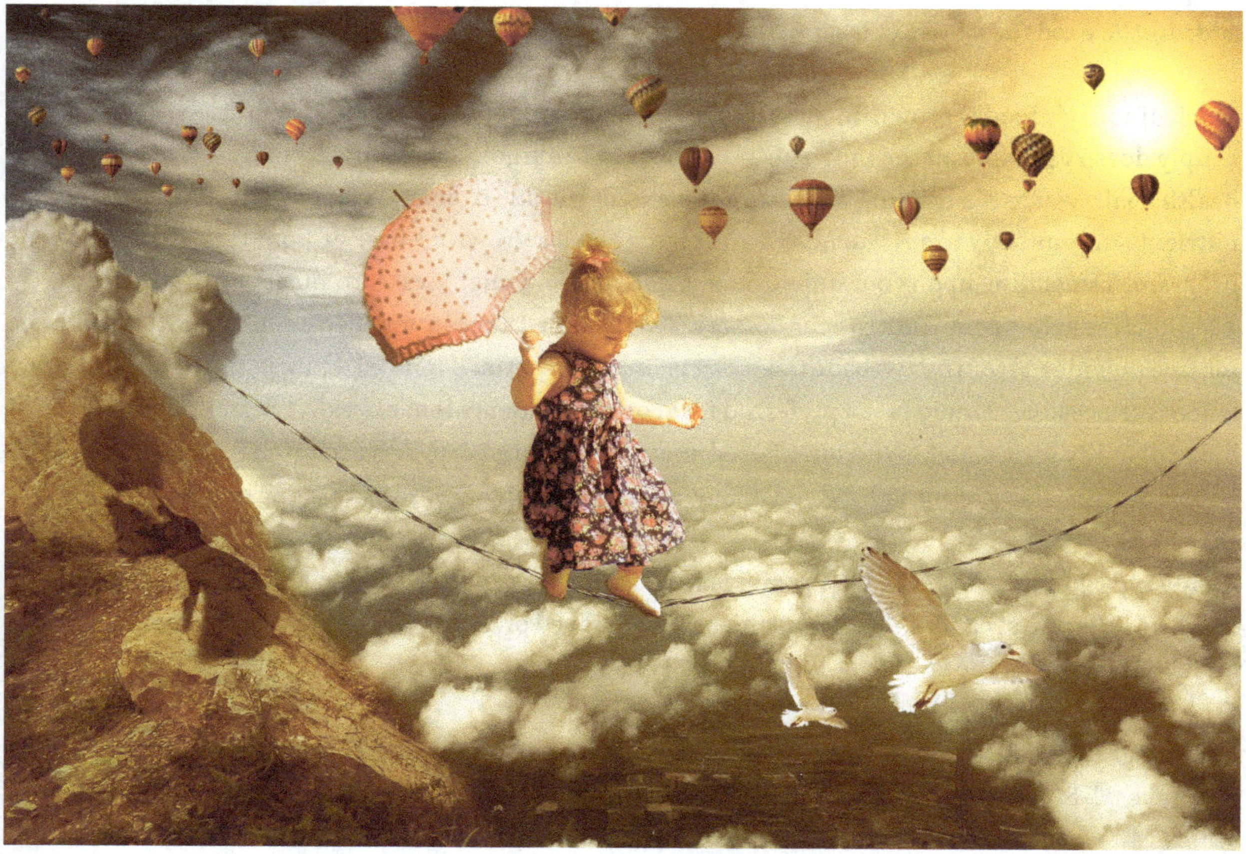

Your Supplement Routine

Yes, I realize supplements aren't sexy. But they can sure help a body become shiny & seem sexy! No matter what your goal was for having surgery, I guarantee you health and energy were part of it. Weight loss doesn't automatically accomplish this. If you're in this for the long haul, you HAVE to address the need for nutritional supplements.

Much of today's food is grown on massive factory farms under less than ideal conditions. The soil simply doesn't provide all the nutrients we need. The same goes for animal farms. To achieve your health goals, you're likely going to need a supplement routine to ensure you have the levels of micro-nutrients in your body to sustain health and vigor. You'll start with a base of liquid vitamins in this program. Depending upon your unique medical issues, you might want to consider expanding to additional supplements. Talk to your doctors. I've included a recommended supplement list available for free download from our website (www.bariatricketo.com). You'll notice I've included liquid vitamins whenever possible. Liquid is the preferred form of supplements that offers WLSers the highest bioavailability of product. With our altered anatomy, pills and capsules can often pass through our bodies only partially absorbed. So you're paying for something you're just peeing out.

Candy type gummies are NEVER a good idea. Those babies can pack a mean amount of carbs – as much as a Starburst candy! The supplements are sprayed on at the end of the manufacturing process and often rub off in the jar.

Nasal is great – however not many supplements are available via that route. If you're offered nasal B12, take it! Sublingual supplements (melt in your mouth) often have fillers and sugars added, which can add carbs.

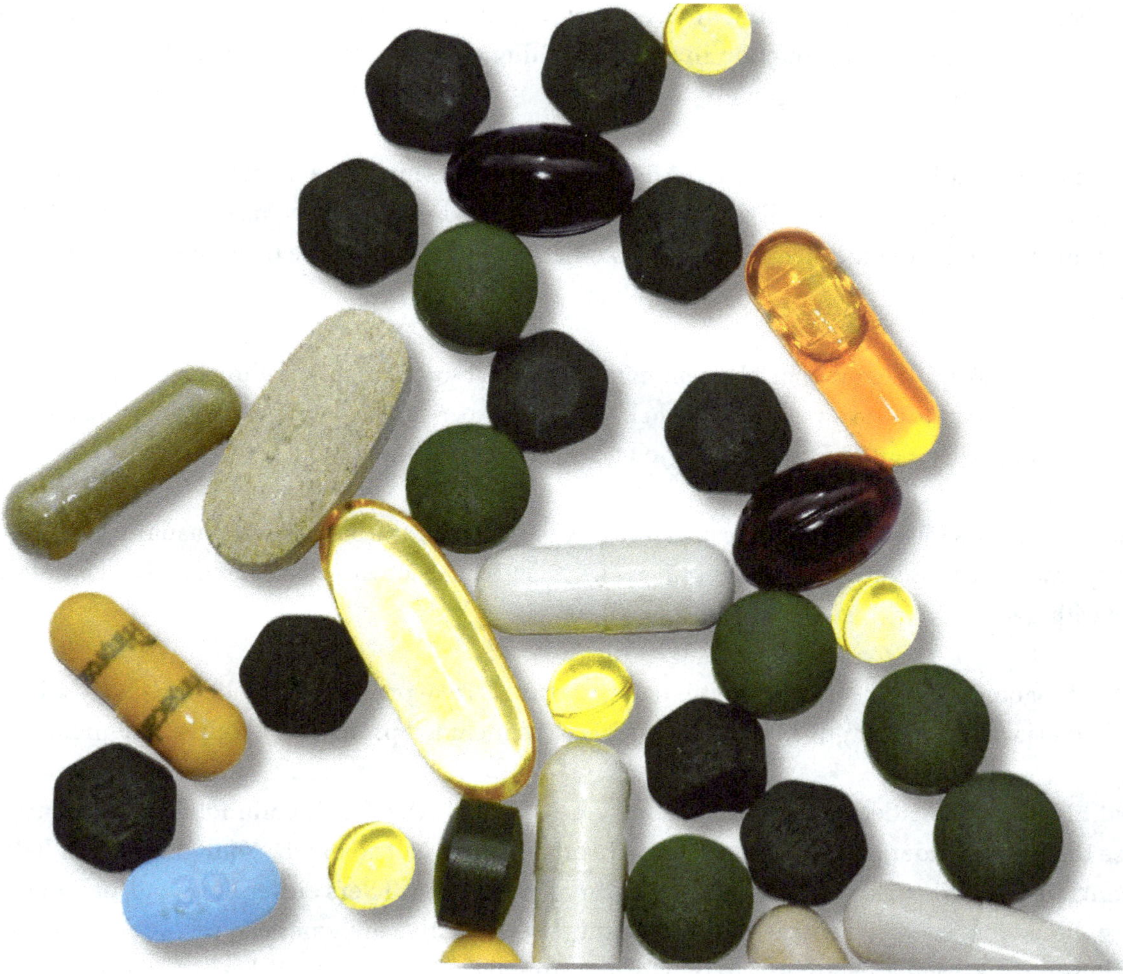

ALWAYS BUY THE BEST SUPPLEMENTS YOU CAN AFFORD – but – highest priced doesn't always mean the best for our non-mainstream bodies. Choose wisely.

Want to keep your hair? Consume protein rather than supplement with Biotin. The National Institute of Health (NIH) has issued warnings to doctor's offices and labs regarding the effect Biotin can have in skewing serum (blood) tests. Everything in the human body is comprised of protein. Adequate consumption of protein is one of the easiest things you can do to insure health. However – like everything, protein can be overdone. Excess protein is stored as fat by the body. Thus the need for you to eat to your own individual protein level. Protein is one of the macros you'll be assigned by your trainer in your individual training. They will review your individual history and conditions to determine your macro levels.

Neurologists stand by zinc, selenium and copper for WLS patients. Joint juice, rich in glucosamine, often provides a significant reduction in pain for aching spines and joints. Liquid forms are best and are included in our supplement guide.

Problems in the bathroom department? Add calcium/magnesium to get things moving. Just make sure to add both – otherwise you'll throw off the body's ratios of these two minerals. Again, the highest bioavailability comes from liquid supplements. Our favorites are included in the supplement guide.

Remember your skin is a semipermiable membrane. You can absorb magnesium through an epsom salt bath. With 1 cup of Epsom Salts in a very warm bath. If you don't experience a bowel movement within an hour, add another cup. Use as much Epsom Salt as you like.

Tendency towards UTIs? Regular use of cranberry extract (not the sugary juice) usually keeps urinary tract infections at bay. The active ingredient is D-Mannose. This an be purchased as a powder& mixed with water.

Bloated? A good probiotic will eliminate that in no time! Take probiotics just before bed to allow the good bacteria to sit in your gut as long as possible. I've included probiotics in our supplement guide.

No gallbladder? Consider taking digestive enzymes. Outside the US it's common for doctors to advise their gallbladder patients to use them. Inside the US? Not so much. Your gallbladder helps concentrate your bile to break down fat. An estimated 80% of WLSers either have had, or will have, their gallbladders removed within 1 year post-surgery. Digestive enzymes can replace most of the functions of this organ. They come in two forms, animal & plant based. We've included this in our supplement guide.

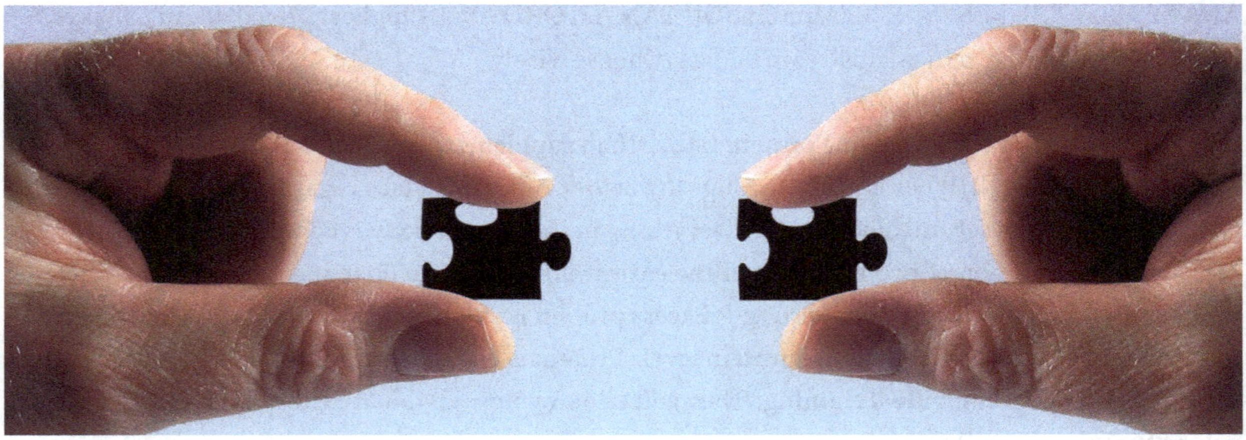

"Your positive action combined with positive thinking results in success."
~Shiv Khera

General Issues

Want to keep your teeth? Don't forget mouth health. Dental problems plague many WLSers starting around 1 year post surgery. GERD issues are common among the weight loss surgery community. Letting these issues go uncontrolled can result in throat and mouth issues. But even those who have had zero mouth issues in the past can suddenly find they are needing restorations, crowns and implants. Head it off by using Biotene for reduced salivation which can leave teeth dry and susceptible to germs. Increase your brushing to after every meal. Carry a toothbrush for this purpose. If your jaw hurts in the morning, consider having a mouth guard made. Most dental insurance covers them. No dental insurance? Buy a boil & mold guard over the counter or invest in having a custom guard made by your dentist. They are MUCH less expensive than restorations. Let your dentist know you've had weight loss surgery. Dentists are trained to look for small changes they might otherwise disregard in the general public. They might advise you to see your GI doc. Restoration dental work is very expensive and often avoidable.

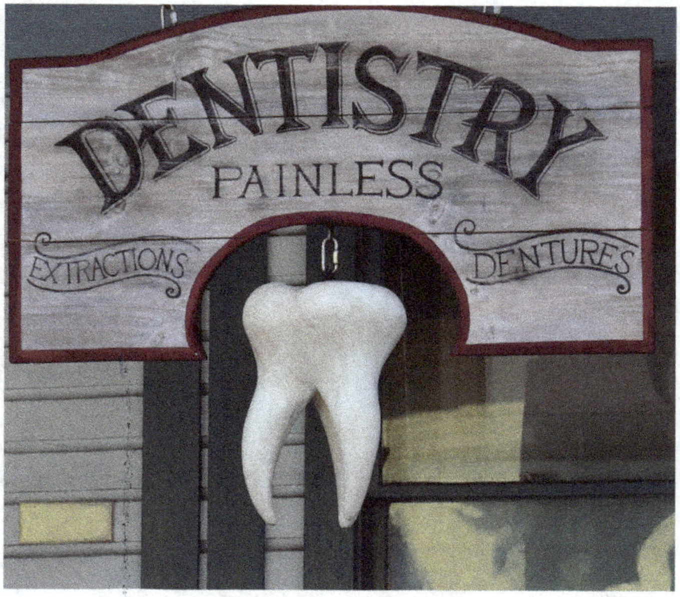

Depression, anxiety and thyroid issues are very real symptoms of the majority of our community. This includes PCOS. My personal belief is they are controlled in the gut. Recent scientific findings seem to be validating this theory. When our gut flora goes bonkers our hormones go along for the ride, creating the effect of insulin resistance or metabolic syndrome. Never hesitate to ask your doctor about any of these conditions or anything else you're experiencing. Chances are they've seen the issue in other WLSers and can help with your symptoms. Remember, you HAVE to be your own advocate. If your doctor isn't familiar with WLS issues, ask to be referred to one that is. You can always use our Facebook groups to network and find a professional in your area.

Feeling tired, dragging & headaches? Ask your doctor to order a metabolic panel complete with inverse thyroid functions showing free T3 and T4. Have your iron & B vitamin levels checked. Thyroid issues and both iron & pernicious anemia are common ailments in our population. Please note: A simple metabolic panel Does Not meet these needs.

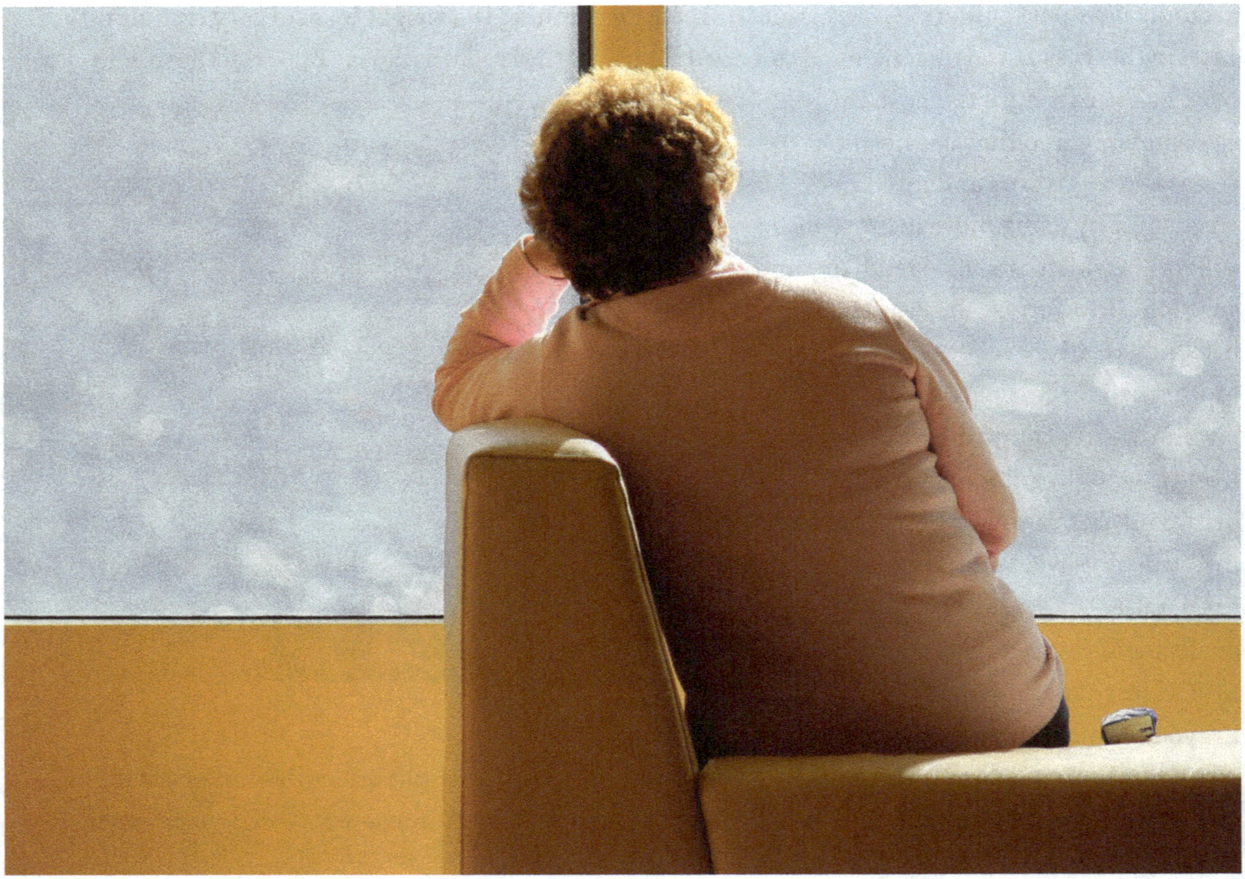

 Content provided in this book is of a general nature only and does not replace the information and advice provided by your own health care professionals. Always consult your own health care providers for specific personal health and medical advice.

2

What is ReStart?

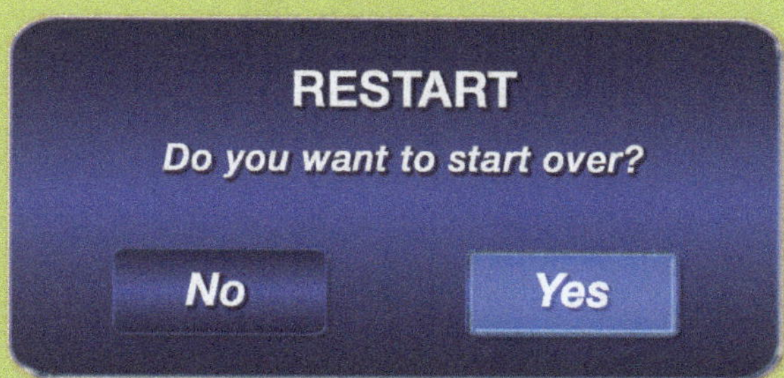

Remember the stomach restriction you felt post-surgery? You can get that back by following ReStart. No, it does not take the place of a revision surgery or shrink a stretched stomach. Only more surgery can do that. Most of us simply need to re-find our point of satiety. It's the point where we're satisfied with the amount we've eaten, but not yet FULL. We could eat one more bite, but it would likely make us uncomfortable both with the pressure it exerts and the knowledge we are out eating our surgery. ReStart is NOT a return to protein powders or mushy baby food. Such diets don't work long term for the simple reason they are boring and usually end in bingeing on old favorite foods.

When you go through ReStart your body will get used to being satisfied with less food. Your stomach contracts and restriction is restored. Weight is lost without that terrible gnawing hunger. You haven't changed your stomach size. You simply reset your satiety point.

TRUTH: Going back to eating like you did just after surgery is dumb. Baby food and a BRAT diet can only get you so far. Eating clean nutritious food will get you healthy.

TRUTH: Most protein powders and shakes taste like crap. Those that do taste decent are usually high in carbs or full of chemicals. If you can't pronounce the ingredients on the label, you don't want it in your body. Ingredients like Splenda and carrageenan hold back weight loss.

YOU HAVE TO MAKE THE DECISION
TO LOSE WEIGHT IN YOUR HEAD

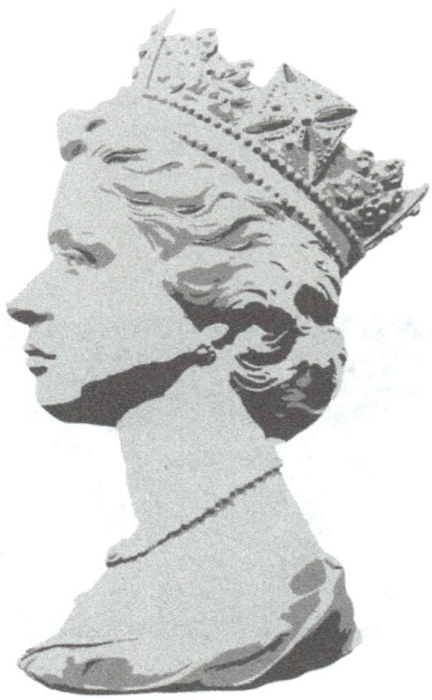

NOT YOUR STOMACH

-Jean Nidetch

TRUTH: Sooner or later, EVERY WLSer is going to need ReStart. It doesn't matter if you're at goal weight and want to stay there, need to lose the last stubborn 20 pounds, or shed the regain weight. Eventually everyone who has weight loss surgery needs ReStart. It's another tool in your weight loss kit. Many members will use ReStart repeatedly prior to achieving goal weight.

TRUTH: It isn't healthy to stay on the ReStart program indefinitely. The program doesn't provide the long term balanced nutrition your body requires to stay healthy. It's a GREAT tool - but not a long term solution. That's what our menu app is for. Please allow a minimum of 4 weeks before going through ReStart again.

Each time you go through the program you'll gain new insights into the reasons why you over eat and mindful coping skills. As your weight goes down, your confidence level goes up. Soon you'll find yourself applying the mindfulness techniques to other areas of your life.

FULL SIGNALS

Everyone's full signal is a bit different. Chances are you've already encountered and know yours. For me, I get sense of slight pressure in my stomach. If I take 1 more bite, my nose starts to run. If I take a second bite, I feel a painful amount of pressure internally that I wouldn't wish on my worst enemy. Some people burp, others hiccup. Many start salivating profusely. Whatever your full signal is – listen to it! That signal is going to get you to and keep you at goal weight!

Want to keep that same satiety point after ReStart? NEVER take "one last bite" after receiving your full signal.

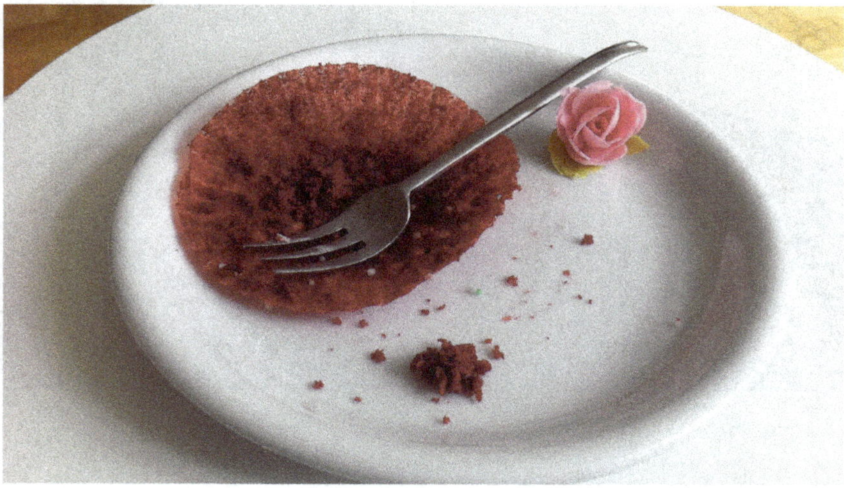

2

How does the Program Work & Who is it For?

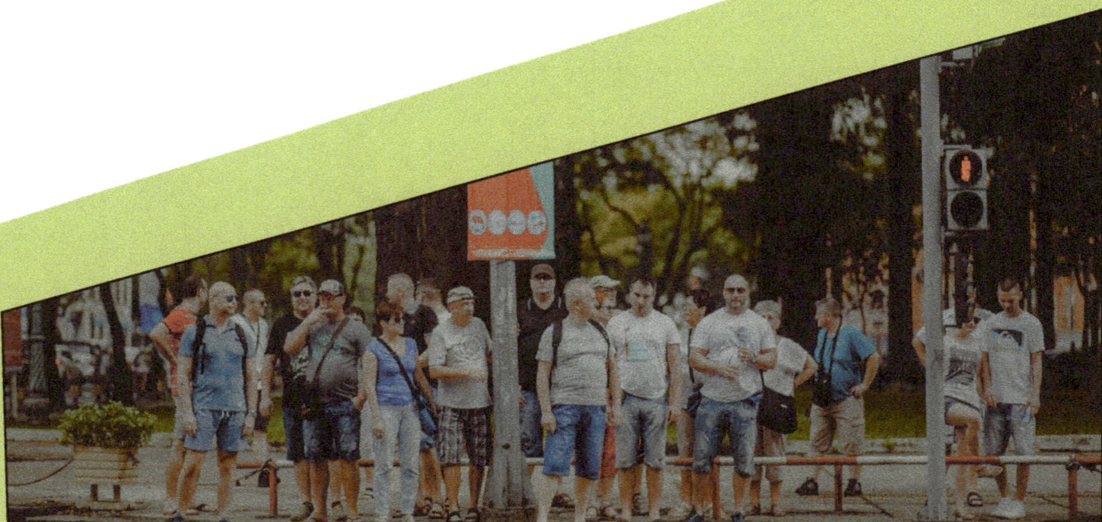

Content provided in this book is of a general nature only and does not replace the information and advice provided by your own health care professionals. Always consult your own health care providers for specific personal health and medical advice.

ReStart was designed to help the "slow losers" - those who have had a hard time losing weight after WLS. If you're at least 3 months post-surgery, and have:

- Experienced a weight loss stall of more than 2 weeks
- Found goal weight out of reach despite sticking to a serious eating regimen
- Consumed over 35 carbs on a daily basis
- Regained weight
- Decided to start modified Keto post WLS and need to detox

Then this is the program for you!

ReStart is a 14-day mindfulness and weight loss program. You'll learn new strategies to keep you focused and on track to goal weight; and you'll achieve your goal weight in a healthy manner that you'll be able to maintain for life.

Days 1 – 4 take you into ketosis and restart the weight loss process.
Days 5 – 9 show you how to incorporate healthy eating and mindfulness into your days.
Days 10 – 14, the end of ReStart, begin your transition into the BariKeto style of eating. It's the perfect time to receive training in our ways and start to use our menu app.

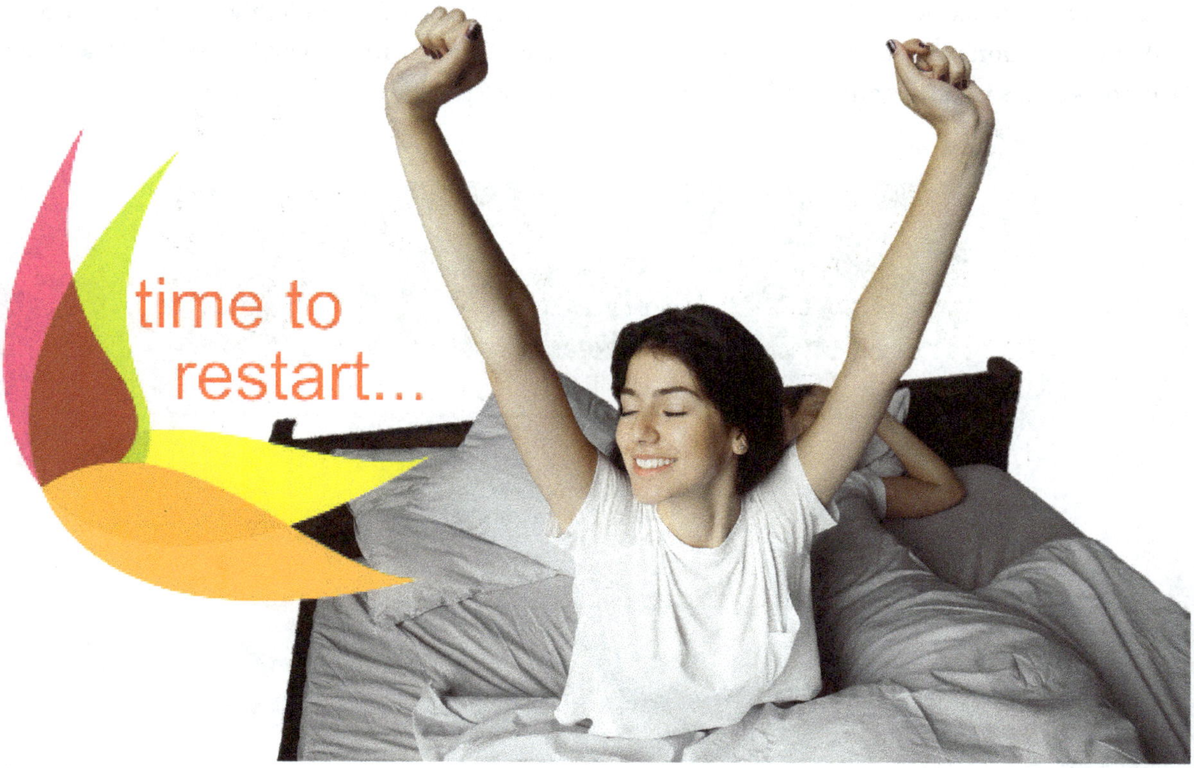

KETOSIS

It's a word you're going to hear A LOT around here. According to medical literature, ketosis is a normal metabolic process. When the body does not have enough glucose for energy, it burns stored fats instead; this results in a build-up of acids called ketones within the body. Some people, like us, encourage ketosis by following a diet called the ketogenic or low-carb diet. It takes the fat we have so much of and turns it into energy. We become fat burning machines!

Please note, Ketosis DOES NOT lead to ketoacidosis. Ketoacidosis is completely different. It occurs in diabetics who don't take their insulin, or sick people who are starving. It can be deadly. If someone tells you ketosis is dangerous, they are likely confusing the two terms.

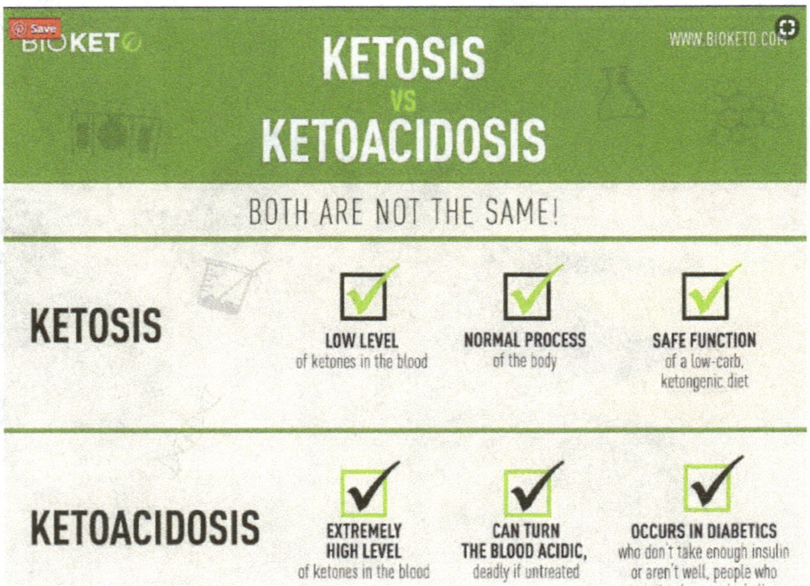

The majority of WLSers have some level of metabolic resistance due to excess carbohydrate intake. This alone makes weight loss and maintenance difficult. Add to it data that says many WLS patients have elevated blood glucose levels and may suffer from glycemic events such as hyperglycemia. To combat blood sugar swings & the feeling of weakness, many turn to carb consumption. It's the DEAD WRONG solution that leaves you fat and exhausted.

HOW LONG DOES IT TAKE TO GET INTO KETOSIS?

How fast you enter ketosis is entirely dependent upon the rate your body clears the excess sugar from your system. Cheat and you just set yourself back. Members of BariKeto report lessened cravings, greater focus, more energy, a sense of well-being and a rate of weight loss they were previously unable to sustain.

Keto Flu: It's an unpleasant title for your body's transition from using sugar to using fat for fuel. There's absolutely NO REASON to suffer through keto flu. The transition from carbs to fat usually takes 2 – 3 days. During this time your body can feel "off". You may experience a stuffy head, dizziness, weakness, headache, or just achy. Simply take some Tylenol, drink some pickle juice, or suck on some pink Himalayan salt. My go-to is Ultima flavored water. It's a powdered mix high in electrolytes that comes in a range of flavors. As WLSers we tend not to mix the drink as strong, so a single canister lasts a long time.

YOU'RE GOING TO WAR

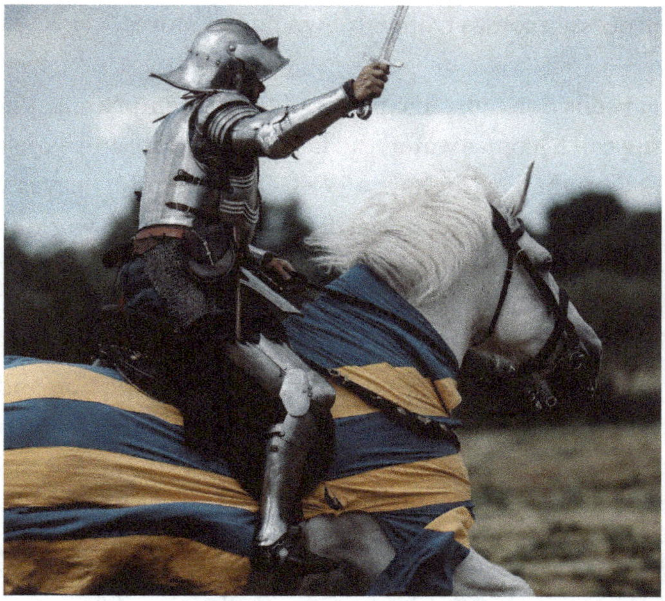

To be effective in the war you're about to enter, you first need to understand a few ground rules. Like all battle strategies, I'm going to give you a high-level snapshot of the playing field. There's a lot more involved than the simplistic overview here. But for most people, this is all you'll need to know.

When the body senses sugar it releases insulin. The insulin directs the sugar to where it is needed in the body. If none of the body's processes need it, the sugar is stored for later use. Carbs cause a large insulin response. Protein causes a smaller

insulin response. Fat causes almost no insulin response.
The more carbs we consume, the more insulin we produce. Do this enough and eventually our bodies quit producing the insulin we need to bring our blood sugar levels back to normal. This is Type 2 diabetes.

Your body likes the status quo. It wants things to continue as normal, even if that normal is detrimental to your health. Your body likes the current level of carbs you're ingesting. When you cut back, and your blood sugar levels are no longer elevated, initially your body will cause you to crave carbs. This is where your battle begins. More carbs = more fat.

Hold fast during cravings. Don't give into the skirmish going on in your body. For each skirmish you win the subsequent skirmishes (cravings) will be reduced in intensity. But give in just once and you're back to your original starting point with cravings.

Studies have shown Keto is an excellent tool for managing, and in some cases, reversing type 2 diabetes. Hypoglycemic events are minimized when following a keto protocol, however, mainstream keto isn't appropriate for a WLS body. Due to our altered anatomy, and many times a lack of gallbladder, when we eat large amounts of fat nasty consequences take place. They range from gas and IBS to gallstones and even removal of the few gallbladders left among us. Sounds gross, but it can be quite painful and even deadly.

Bariatric Keto says, "Why add a lot of fat if my body already has plenty?" We advocate eating a moderate amount of fat. Just enough to get into ketosis. The remainder of the fat needed for bodily processes comes from our own body's stores.

Fat cells don't just disappear when they empty out. They initially fill with water. When enough of the cell becomes water, the fat cell contracts and expels the water. This is known as a WHOOSH. Overnight you can have a WHOOSH that often leaves you 2 – 3 pounds (.91 - 1.36 kg) lighter. No, you didn't lose that much overnight. You had been working towards the weight loss by replacing the fat in the cell with water. When people say, "it's just water weight" I don't think they realize that weight used to be fat. The key to starting a WHOOSH is water and potassium/electrolytes.

Fat is required for proper nervous system function and is essential in the production of hormones. Fat coats nerve endings and dulls the body's pain signals to the brain. And fat truly is where the flavor is. Low fat foods taste like cardboard before all the chemical crap is added.

When blood sugar is stabilized, ketosis helps promote hormone regulation which results in better sleep, increased energy, mood stabilization. It's even shown a positive impact on menstrual regulation.

We encourage ketosis because we want to lose excess weight and gain better overall health. Consuming a moderate amount of fat helps us attain ketosis, distribute nutrition through the body and is far more satisfying to consume than a bland shake diet. Fat keeps you full between feedings.

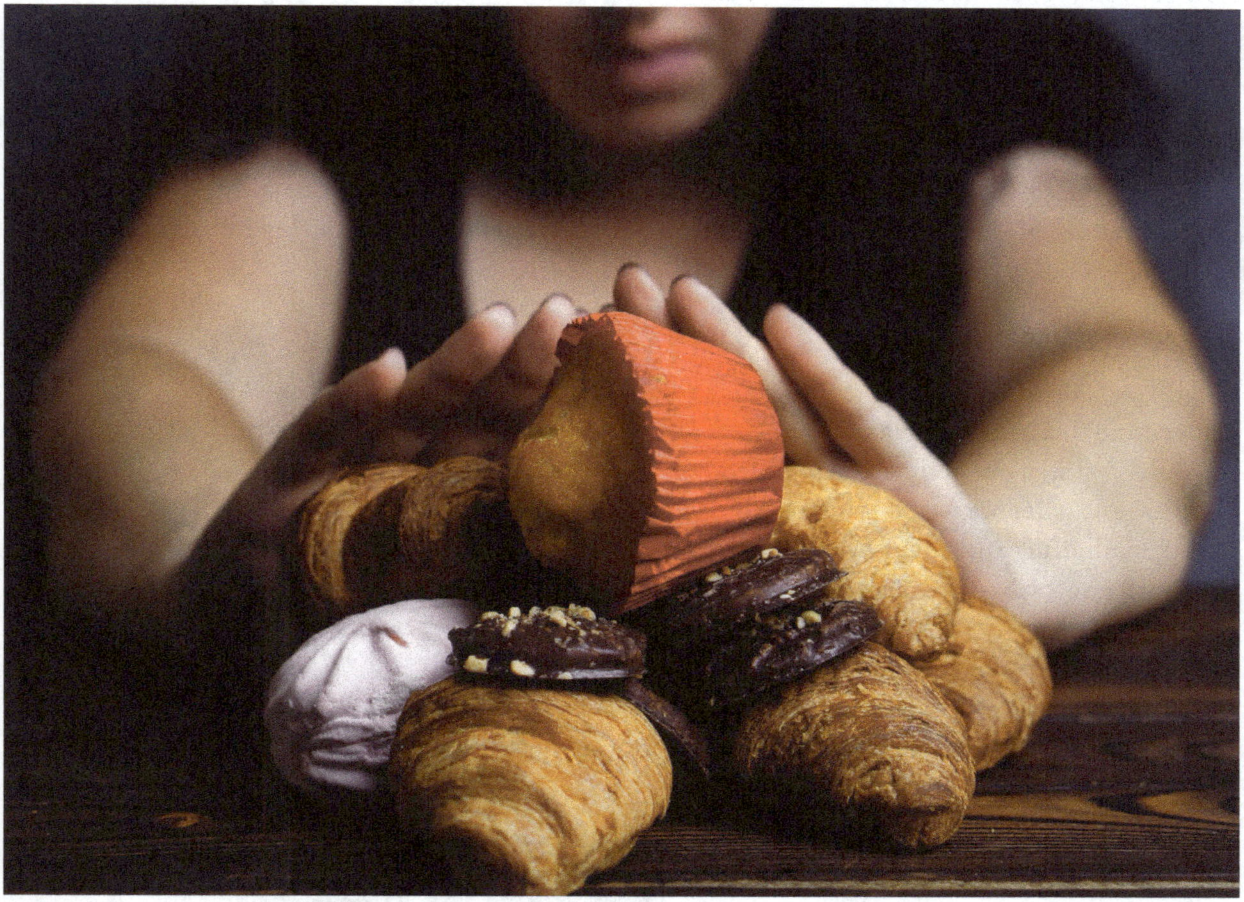

THIS IS A CARB WAR

Carbohydrates must be limited in order to lose weight through ketosis. Your body is a well-oiled machine. Its preferred energy source is carbs. In order to switch your body's energy source to fat, you're going to be required to restrict carb intake.

Now food manufacturers would like you to believe carbs – fiber – sugar alcohols = net carbs.
Net carbs was a theory put forward by a researcher once in a white paper. The food industry grabbed onto it with both hands as a way to make diet foods taste decent. Suddenly a new "diet" industry

sprang up touting their products would help you lose weight. Problem was, they didn't. Even the FDA realized they didn't and doesn't allow the manufacturers to say they are a diet food. That protein bar you ate yesterday? It was most likely roughly equivalent nutritionally to a candy bar. The researcher did come back and recant the theory of net carbs, but by then the genie was out of the bottle. Recently New York state sued the makers of "diet soda" saying their products are anything but diet. Don't fall for the hype. There is no such thing as net carbs. A carb is a carb.

HOWEVER, not all carbs are created equal. A simple carb, such as a candy bar, doesn't hold the nutritional value of a complex carbohydrate. For the purposes of this program we are going to largely treat all carbs the same. Just know, in the back of your mind, your mom was right. Veggies are good for you. Again, some have better nutritional values than others. But veggies are carbs. We simply limit our intake of them while in the weight loss phase. We get them back during carb cycling and at maintenance when we've achieved goal weight.

FEED ME, SEYMOUR!

Understand that hunger pangs are a physiological sign our body needs to be fed. But what and when we feed it is up to us. Through mindful eating habits you're going to relearn how to interpret those hunger pangs.

Most of us have never truly experienced hunger. Sure, we've been hungry. But true hunger is rare in our daily lives. "Am I truly hungry, or is this head hunger?" is a question you'll learn to ask yourself often.

I think of it like this – imagine your worst, most hated food of all time. Now imagine it smooshed with dirt on it. Are you interested in eating it? You would be if you were truly hungry. Anything else is head hunger.

Mindful eating gives you back the controller. You, not your body, determine what and how much you consume. That control enables you to get to goal weight – and stay there!

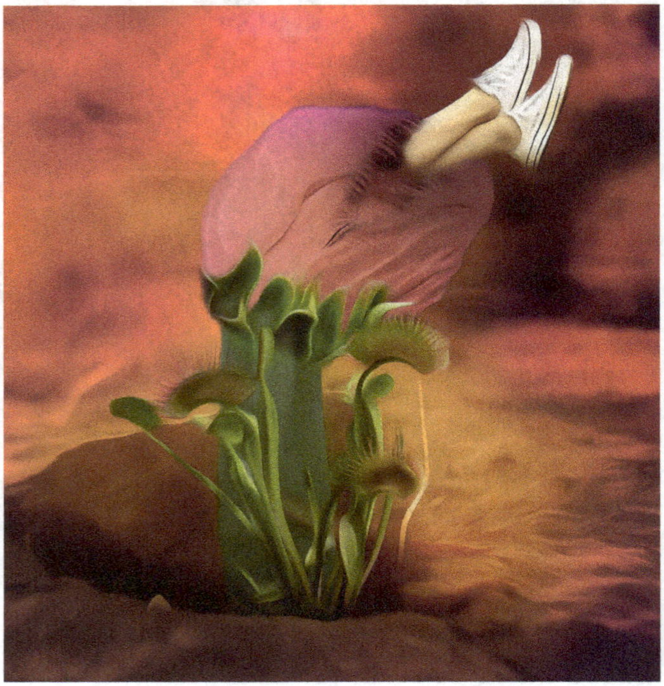

Nights are always hard. My monsters come out from under the bed and make themselves known. Dreams bring insight and peace. Mornings brings hope and sometimes strength to try again.

-- Mary Beth Filer

HEY, SEYMOUR. MEET INTERVAL FASTING!

Want fewer cravings? Interval Fasting is the quickest way to overcome head hunger. Your body knows when it can expect to be fed, and when food will not be offered. The brain quickly adapts and stops expending energy to produce cravings to try to get you to eat. It also allows your body's digestive system to rest from food intake during "off hours".

Begin with an 8 hour eating window. Don't like breakfast? Don't eat it. I begin my eating window at 11 am and end at 7 pm. I find I want to eat more at night. You may be the opposite. You may need that breakfast muffin to help with the morning commute. Try different 8 hour eating windows and see what works best for you. If necessary you can always extend the eating window to 10 hours.

Anything under 50 calories doesn't break your fast. That's 50 calories TOTAL through the fast. So a cup of caffeine in the morning to bring you alive is fine. It's what you put in the caffeine that can break your fast. Be mindful of what you add and stay within BariKeto food guidelines. I like stevia and powdered MCT oil in my caffeine to start my day.

YOUR SECRET WEAPON - EXOGENOUS KETONES

Exogenous means anything made outside of the body. You already know what ketones are. I've experienced an easier time getting into, and staying in, ketosis by using certain exogenous ketones. The energy boost is amazing, and they usually taste pretty darn good. But, like most industries, you can get caught overpaying for hype. Everything from big food manufacturers to MLM organizations have entered this market. I've included them in your beginning days to give you a boost during fasting. You may choose to continue their usage or not - the decision is yours to make based on the benefit (or non-benefit) you derive from them. There's no reason to spend a fortune on them. Just make sure they are sweetened with stevia ONLY and contain few carbs.

If you're around the keto community very long, you'll see the crap storm the term exogenous ketones elicits. Some swear by them. Others call them expensive urine. Whatever camp you end up in, remember these things:

- What works for you may not work as well for someone else, and vise-versa. No one product has the same effect on everyone. Your mileage may vary.
- They are chock full of quick releasing B & D vitamins that can help you power through a tough period of time.
- You can get caffeinated or uncaffeinated - your choice. If you choose caffeinated make sure you

add it to your day's total caffeine intake. I get uncaffeinated & have a canister of caffeine that I draw from if I want the drink caffeinated.

- They helps you get the electrolytes your body needs.

Caveat: I've yet to find an exogenous ketone that didn't taste like crap without flavoring. Manufacturers mask the taste using citric acid for flavor. Too much citric acid can burn our new stomachs and cause ulcers. Consider halving the recommended serving size in order to dilute the taste and citric acid concentration.

THE BATTLE PLAN

Great battle plans often consist of a pincer movement – two active plans to attack and pin the enemy. The first is clean mindful eating. The second is supplementation. BOTH are necessary to achieve goal weight and health.

You have two options in your battle plan. One has 2 days of liquids prior to eating food again. The second has 3 days of liquids. Both get you to the same place. Both are the ReStart program. The first plan starts slower, with a gradual slide into ketosis and 2 days of liquids. The second begins fast with 3 days of liquids. Which option you choose to follow this time, or subsequent times through the program, depends entirely on you. I will give you one piece of food for thought to consider when choosing. If you have trouble stopping eating once you start, you might find the first day liquids only the easier option. That's me. If food isn't around, and I know I'm not going to get it that day, I'm OK with that once I tell my body NO a few times. However, once I start eating, I don't want to stop. It's like someone opened the barn door and let the animals escape. Others are more disciplined and don't need as strict of an approach.

EVERY night & morning you'll take your liquid supplements. You'll soon find you have more energy, enjoy taking fewer pills, and spend less on them than the individual supplements you were purchasing. Please note some liquid supplements require refrigeration. I refrigerate the vitamins, cal/mag and joint juice. Only the minerals are shelf stable at room temperature once opened.

These next two parts may sound hokey and new agey. I'm a HUGE skeptic of anything I can't quantify. Give me hard data or I won't believe what you're saying. However - for whatever reason - these have worked for so many of us that I can't deny the success rates. Each does have science to back it up. But the science is neurology based and can get pretty high level for us mere mortals. I've included references in the Appendix for those that are interested in exploring the rationale behind them.

EVERY morning you'll be greeting the sun for 15 - 20 minutes with a bare face and without sunglasses.

Ideally with bare feet in the grass. This doesn't mean stare into the sun. Please don't. Simply enjoy the display of changing colors and light as the sun rises. If your sunrise is cold, bundle up. But do not cover your face or eyes. In fact, if it's warm, the less you wear the more benefit you'll derive. Sunlight helps determine the structure of the mitochondria in your body as well as reset your circadian rhythm. Our ancestors developed on this planet and our bodies have evolved to be tied to its rhythms. If you work third shift, try to greet the sun rise when you're getting off.

If you're exposed to electronic screens all day, such as computer screens, consider a screen to block the blue light. I used to experience fatigue and headaches at the end of each day. My husband purchased an inexpensive pair of yellow tinted blue light blocking glasses for me on Amazon. I was skeptical, but figured all I had to lose was my vanity because they looked dorky. To my surprise, after a few days I actually noticed a difference at night if I had warn the glasses that day. Vanity won, however, and I switched to hard molded plastic tinted screens that I now use religiously. They sit over my monitors on my desktop & laptop and are actually far more effective at headache and eye fatigue reduction than the glasses were. But again, I was using cheap glasses. I'm told there are better ones available that don't have a yellow tint and make you look dorky. Some prescription glasses manufacturers are even offering it as an option.

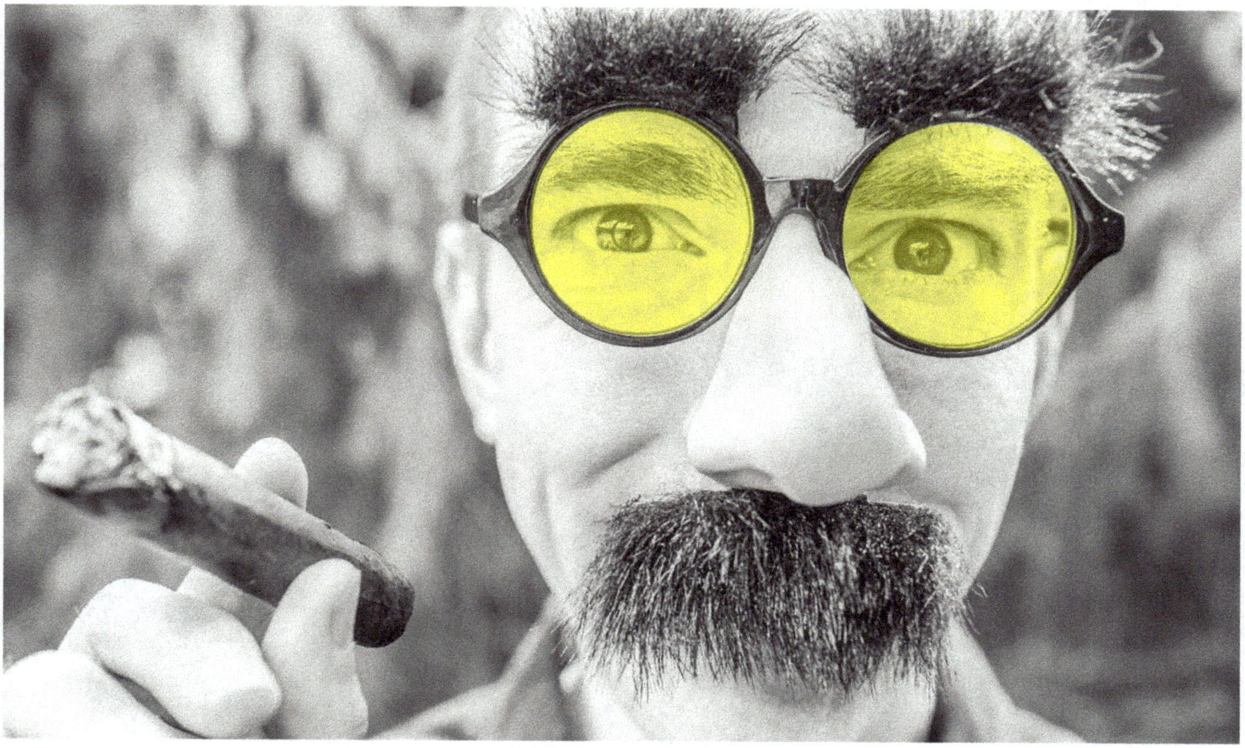

A few interesting facts:
Approximately 95% of Serotonin is in our GI tract – not our brain. Researchers have linked mental disorders to gut biome. It's reasonable to believe "fixing" our gut biome can fix far more than just obesity level.

When you eat something pleasurable, the feeling is stored as data in our brains in the same region our fondest memories are stored. Food colors our perception of the world around us, our hormone production and our cellular health.

Deriving pleasure from eating is completely natural. However, those feelings do us no favors when fighting obesity. It's too easy to fall back into old patterns. The easiest way to cut the emotions from food is to stop intake of food, for a little while! Plus, a short period of fasting permits your body to cease the physical demands of processing food and allows you to concentrate on higher level functions, such as mindful eating and your relationship with food.

Sometimes we should express our gratitude for the small and simple things like the scent of the rain, the taste of your favorite food, or the sound of a loved one's voice.

-- Joseph B. Wirthlin

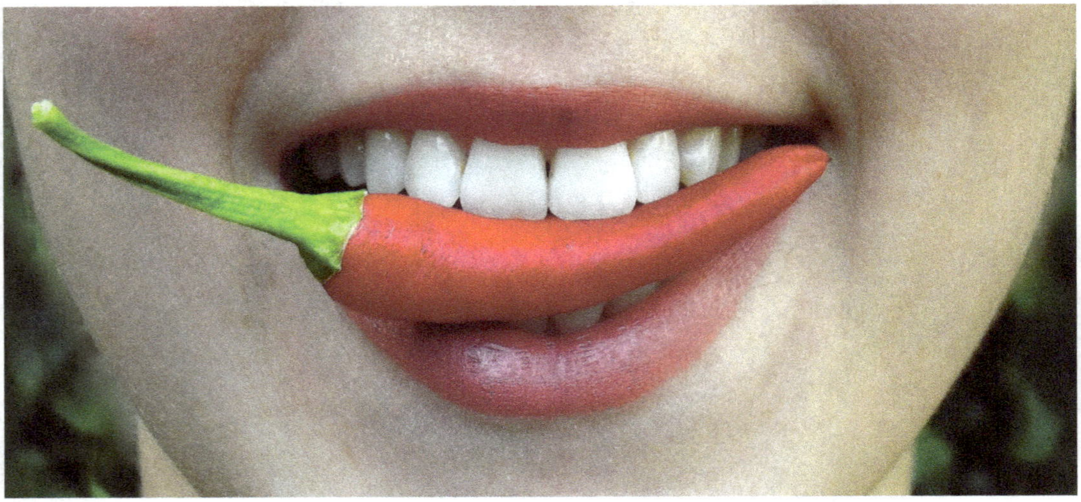

Use this mandala a part of your mindfulness homework throughout your ReStart. Each day color in one layer of the mandala as you practice being present. At the end you will have a work of art to celebrate your success over head hunger.

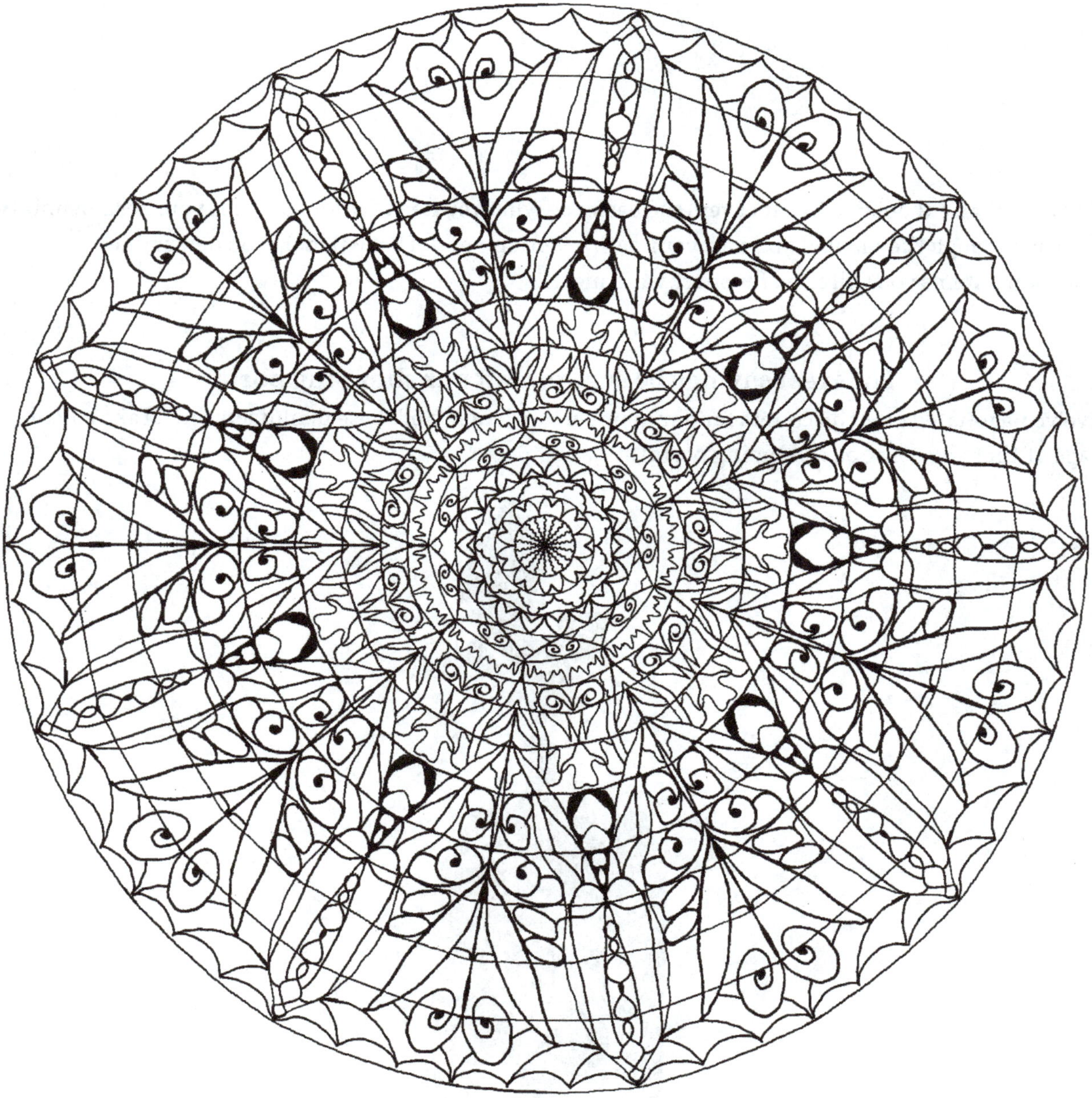

SHOPPING LIST

This is not an exhaustive list. It covers the basics of what you need for ReStart. It is your responsibility to read through the manual and pick your path – Option 1 or 2. That will help you determine additional items you will need for snacks and meals.

For great savings be sure to visit our shopping portal.

We've negotiated great discounts for our members with many of these manufacturers. Take advantage of them by using our shopping portal at www.bariatricketo.com

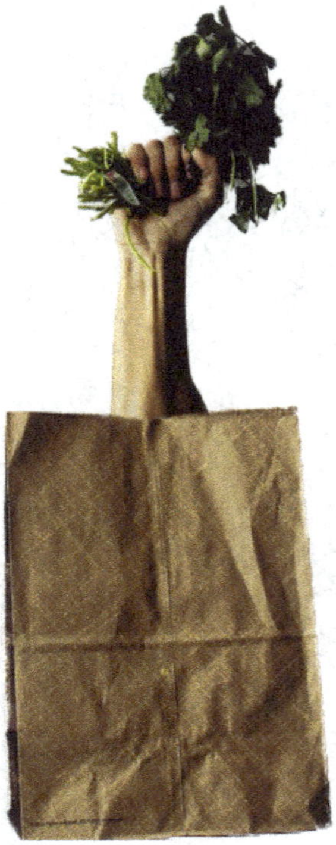

 Content provided in this book is of a general nature only and does not replace the information and advice provided by your own health care professionals. Always consult your own health care providers for specific personal health and medical advice.

- Bragg's Apple Cider Vinegar liquid or any Apple Cider Vinegar capsules WITH the mother.
- Liquid stevia – most prefer Nu Naturals or Sweet Leaf brands
- Herbal tea of your choice WITHOUT sweetener
- Ultima electrolyte enhancer
- Pink Himalayan salt
- Extra virgin light olive oil
- Probiotic with a minimum of 5 different strains·
- Liquid vitamins and supplements. See our free supplement guide on the website for specific manufacturer recommendations
- Broth. No high sodium or MSG. Bone broth is preferred but not required.
  We have lots of recipes if you would likes to make your own!
- 8 – 12 ounces (228 - 336 grams) of dense protein (such as chicken or fish)
- Epsom salt & essential oil of your choice, or just order lavender Epsom Salt.
- Green beans, broccoli, or cauliflower
- Eggs
- NuNaturals Cocoa Syrup (also available in other great flavors)
- Cheddar (not pre-shredded. Get the chunk of cheese) and Feta cheese
- Coconut based lotion and lip balm without petroleum. I like Yes to coconut hand cream and lip balm.
- Exogenous ketones. NutriKeto has a deal on flavored limeade and lemonade that you can get in trial sizes. They do not contain caffeine. If you want to add caffeine, it is available in powder form from stores such as Amazon. Pruvit products are excellent - but very pricey. Please see the shopping portal at www.bariatricketo.com.
- Heavy whipping cream or almond or coconut milk (unflavored & unsweetened) or nut pods. Note: no dairy first few days.
- Coconut Oil·
- Kerry Gold Irish Butter
- Bok Choy, Napa lettuce or Spinach
- Dill Pickles
- Organic Blueberries or Strawberries
- Avocado Mayo or other approved mayo

4

PLAN

I

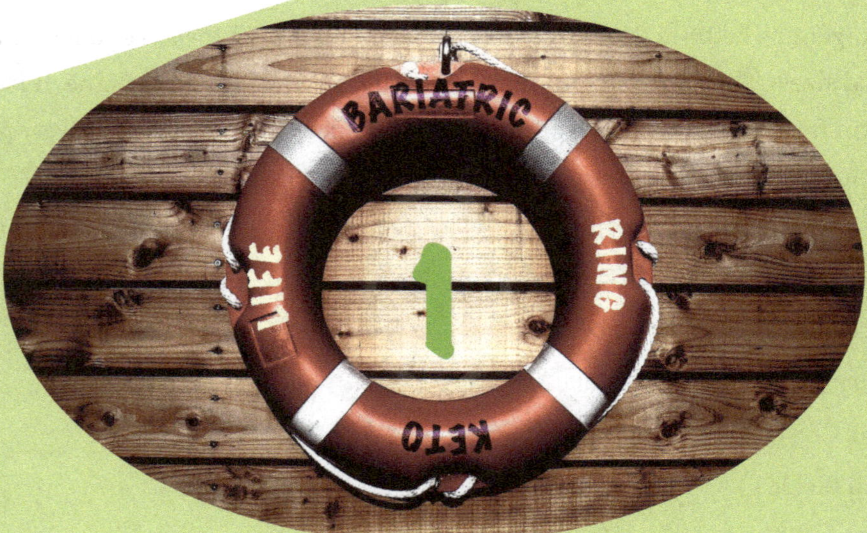

Content provided in this book is of a general nature only and does not replace the information and advice provided by your own health care professionals. Always consult your own health care providers for specific personal health and medical advice.

This is a gentle approach to cleansing your body of toxins and encouraging healing of your gut. Inflammation is naturally controlled when these things happen, often bringing a lessening of pain and emotional relief.

Food intake will cease beginning the prior night no later than 10 pm. Schedule for a day you can concentrate on yourself with few distractions. Don't sabotage yourself by starting on a day with a high stress schedule. Make sure all food shopping has been accomplished prior to starting.

- Days 1 & 2: The first two days of this plan will help you slow down your whirlwind life and get back to the basics. You'll replace chemical filled food with clear liquids in order to encourage the toxins to move out of your body. You'll also be surprised how little food you need to live.
- Days 3 - 5: You'll learn to recognize your full signal as well as your satiety point - and how the two differ.
- Days 6 - 9: With the addition of more food, you'll learn coping mechanisms for FAT HEAD. Now is the time to purchase and schedule 1:1 training so you'll have your macros and be able to transition into our long term eating program.
- Days 8 - the rest of your life: Start with gentle exercises. Gradually increase at your own pace. Remember, exercise only accounts for 20% of weight loss and can actually drive you to consume more. Do it because it makes you feel more alive, lessens depression & anxiety, and helps move water out of your body so you get to experience those wonderful WOOSHes faster!
- Days 10 - 14: Now that you've experienced success with the Bariatric Keto program, you'll prepare to transition to what will become a lifelong way of eating

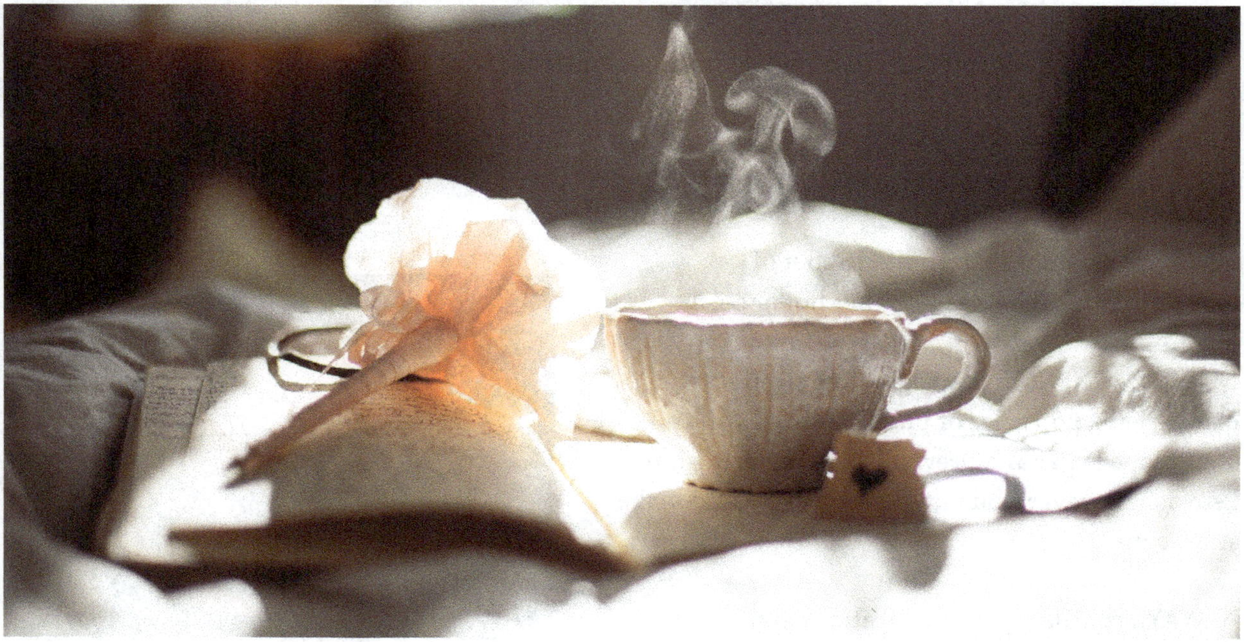

ReStart Plan One - Days 1 & 2

When you wake up, you'll enjoy a cup of hot water + 2 teaspoons (8.5 grams) of ACV (apple cider vinegar) and 1 teaspoon (4.2 grams) of lemon or lime juice.
* If you substitute ACV capsules, make sure they contain "the mother", it's the active ingredient.

Consume your liquid vitamin & minerals. You may consume by shooting or putting in water, coffee, or tea.

Greet the sun for 15 - 20 minutes with a bare face and without sunglasses. Ideally place your bare feet in the grass. Enjoy the dance of colors and the solitude.

Consume up to 2 cups (16 ounces/ 500 ml) of caffeinated beverages throughout the day. Consume black. You may add 1 teaspoon (4.2 grams) of unsweetened almond, coconut milk, or a carb free nut pod if desired, to each cup. Use liquid stevia as a sweetener.

Consume clear liquids only with all solids strained out. Broths such as bone broth, miso soup broth, pho broth, veggie soup broth, etc. Broth must be low sodium and contain no MSG. Limit yourself to 64 fluid ounces (8 cups/1.8 kg) per day.

Prepare and drink one 8 ounce (.23 kg) glass of your preferred flavor of exogenous ketones, with or without caffeine. Do this during your "hump time" when you would normally want to grab a snack to keep going.
Drink at least 72 ounces (2.25 liters) of water throughout the day. Broth counts in this total.

At least 48 ounces (1.42 liters) of the fluid should be electrolyte enhanced. You can use Ultima, pink Himalayan salt, Smart water, etc.

You may consume an unlimited about of uncaffeinated herbal teas - either hot or cold.

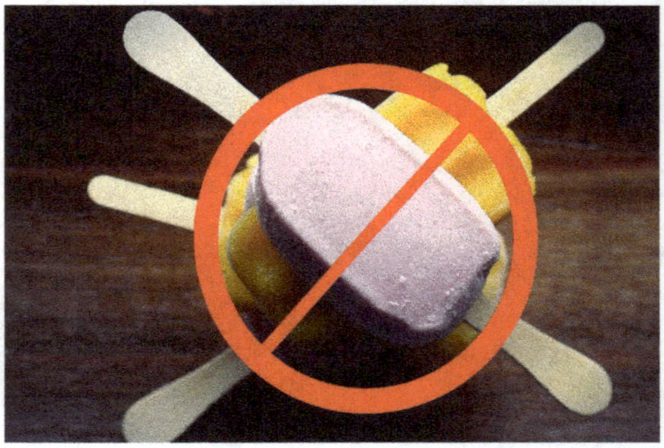

DO NOT CONSUME any sugar-free sweet-tasting drinks, jello, popsicles or pudding. They will spike your blood sugar and prevent you from going into ketosis. However, you may freeze Ultima and make snow cones.

ALWAYS continue your medications and

supplements. End your day by taking your probiotic just prior to going to bed. This will maximize the time it spends in your digestive tract. This is also the time to take your liquid calcium/magnesium in broth, herbal tea, ultima or another liquid.

HINT: If you find plain water boring, try varying the temperature as well as size of ice cubes. You can also use stevia sweetened products ONLY, such as Ultima. No Splenda, sugar, or sugar substitutes except stevia. You may also infuse water with fruit or veggies. You may not, however, consume the veggies or squeeze them.

NOTE: For those with PCOS, thyroid or blood sugar issues, add ½ cup (4 ounces/.11kg) protein of choice and ½ cup non-starchy veggie of choice (total of 1 cup) to the 8 cups of broth on days 1 & 2. You won't lose as much weight, but it will keep you from washing out of the program due to fatigue or dizziness. Be prepared to spend a lot of time running to the toilet.

Food is for eating, and good food is to be enjoyed... I think food is, actually, very beautiful in itself.
--Delia Smith

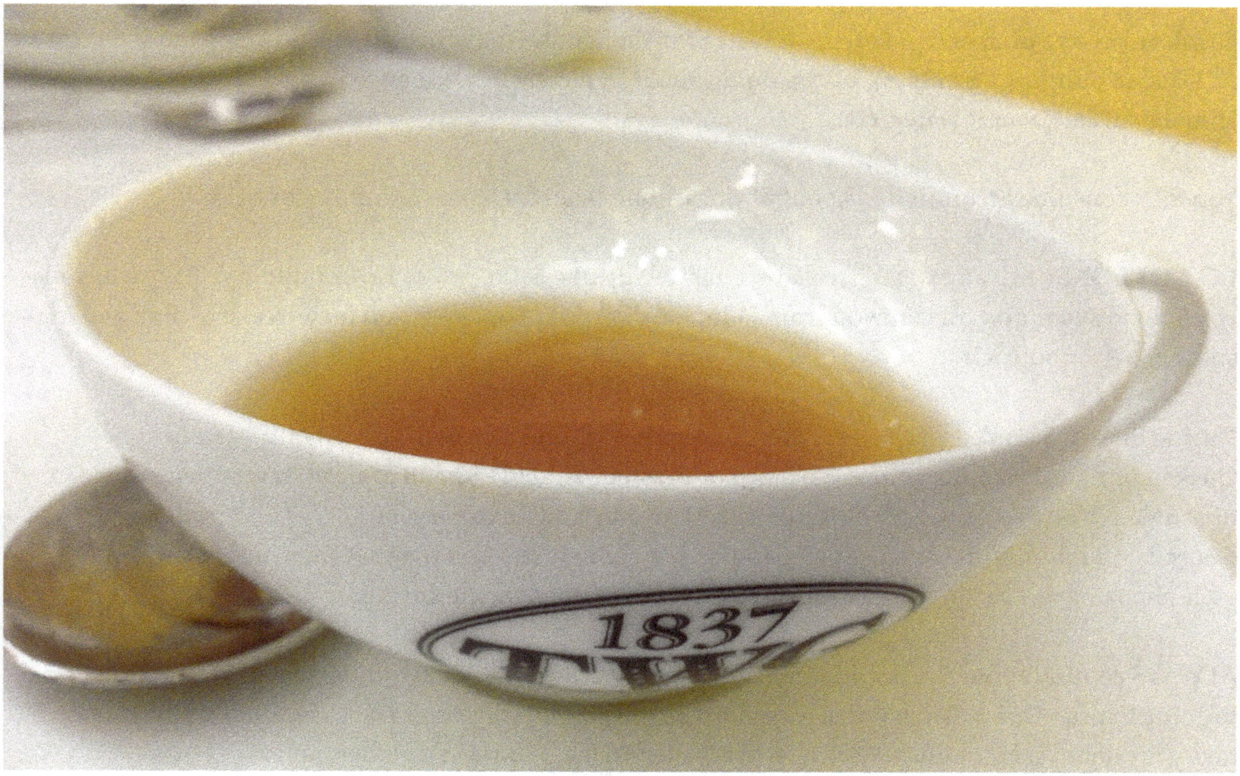

ReStart Plan One Days 3 - 5

When you wake up, you'll enjoy a cup of hot water + 2 teaspoons of ACV (apple cider vinegar) and 1 teaspoon of lemon or lime juice.
* If you substitute ACV capsules, make sure they contain "the mother".

Consume your liquid vitamins & minerals. You may consume by shooting or putting in water, coffee, or tea.

Greet the sun for 15 - 20 minutes with a bare face and without sunglasses. Ideally place your bare feet in the grass. Enjoy the dance of colors and the solitude.
Consume up to 2 cups (16 ounces/ 500 ml) of caffeinated beverages throughout the day. Consume black. You may add 1 teaspoon of unsweetened 1 teaspoon of unsweetened almond, coconut milk, or a carb free nut pod if desired, to each cup. Use liquid stevia as a sweetener.

Continue to consume clear liquids only with all solids strained out. Broths such as bone broth, miso soup broth, pho broth, veggie soup broth, etc. Broth must be low sodium and contain no MSG. Limit yourself to 32 fluid ounces (4 cups) per day.

Drink at least 72 ounces (2.25 liters) of water throughout the day. Broth counts in this total.
At least 48 ounces (1.42 liters) of the fluid should be electrolyte enhanced. You can use Ultima, pink Himalayan salt, Smart water, etc.

You may consume an unlimited about of uncaffinated herbal teas - either hot or cold.

DO NOT CONSUME any sugar-free sweet-tasting drinks, jello, popsicles or pudding. They will spike your blood sugar and prevent you from going into ketosis. However, you may freeze Ultima and make snow cones or popsicles.

During days 3, 4, and 5, you will eat one meal each day. The meal will consist of 2 - 3 ounces of chicken or fish. Prepared grilled, poached or roasted. And ¼ - ½ cup of non-starchy veggies steamed or sautéed in olive oil or apple cider vinegar. You may add 1 teaspoon of Kerry Gold Irish Butter, if desired. Add pink Himalayan sea salt and/or pepper to taste. You may eat this meal at the time of your choosing, however, all of the meal must be consumed in one sitting.

ALWAYS continue your medications and supplements. End your day by taking your probiotic just prior to going to bed. This will maximize the time it spends in your digestive tract. This is also the time to take your liquid calcium/magnesium in broth, herbal tea, Ultima or another liquid.

ReStart Plan One Days 6 - 9

When you wake up, you'll enjoy a cup of hot water + 2 teaspoons of ACV (apple cider vinegar) and 1 teaspoon of lemon or lime juice.
* If you substitute ACV capsules, make sure they contain "the mother".
Consume your liquid vitamins & minerals. You may consume by shooting or putting in water, coffee, or tea.
Greet the sun for 15 - 20 minutes with a bare face and without sunglasses. Ideally place your bare feet in the grass. Enjoy the dance of colors and the solitude.
Consume up to 2 cups (16 ounces/ 500 ml) of caffeinated beverages throughout the day. Consume black. You may add 1 teaspoon of 1 teaspoon of unsweetened almond, coconut milk, or a carb free nut pod if desired, to each cup. Use liquid stevia as a sweetener.

Continue to consume clear liquids with all solids strained out. Broths such as bone broth, miso soup broth, pho broth, veggie soup broth, etc. Broth must be low sodium and contain no MSG. Limit yourself to 16 fluid ounces (2 cups) per day.

Drink at least 72 ounces (2.25 liters) of water throughout the day. Broth counts in this total.
At least 48 ounces (1.42 liters) of the fluid should be electrolyte enhanced. You can use Ultima, pink Himalayan salt, Smart water, etc.

You may consume an unlimited about of caffeine free herbal teas - either hot or cold.

DO NOT CONSUME any sugar-free sweet-tasting drinks, jello, popsicles or pudding. They will spike your blood sugar and prevent you from going into ketosis. However, you may freeze Ultima and make snow cones or popsicles.

Choose ONE one of the following to eat at what would be the beginning of your 8 hour eating window:

1 egg white ONLY (no yoke). Wrap egg white in a napa lettuce leaf (chinese cabbage) with 1 teaspoon of avocado mayo.

6 slices (4 ounces total) of cucumber with 2 tablespoons of feta or cream cheese and 6 almonds

(2) bacon wrapped steamed asparagus spears. Use one slice of bacon per spear.

(3) one ounce of cheddar cheese (28.35 grams).

Choose ONE of the following to eat at what would be the end of your 8 hour eating window:

One large or two small dill pickles with ounce of cheddar cheese (28.33 grams).

10 steamed or raw green string beans (not sugar snap) with 2 teaspoons feta or cream cheese

¼ cup blueberries or sliced strawberries in 1 tablespoon heavy whipping cream

1/2 ounce each of cooked chicken breast and oven roasted ham (not pre-cut sandwich meat) for a total of one ounce of meat.

In addition, consume your meal of 2 - 3 ounces of chicken or fish. Prepared grilled, poached or roasted. And ¼ - ½ cup of non-starchy veggies steamed or sautéed in olive oil or apple cider vinegar. You may add 1 teaspoon of Kerry Gold Irish Butter, if desired. Add pink Himalayan sea salt and/or pepper to taste. You may eat this meal at the time of your choosing, however, all of the meal must be consumed in one sitting.

Days 8 - forever: Resistance bands, walking, yoga, simple stretching, flowing repetitive motion routines like QiGong or Y-Dan. Gradually increase as your weight goes down and stamina goes up.

ALWAYS continue your medications and supplements. End your day by taking your probiotic just prior to going to bed. This will maximize the time it spends in your digestive tract. This is also the time to take your liquid calcium/magnesium in broth, herbal tea, Ultima or another liquid.

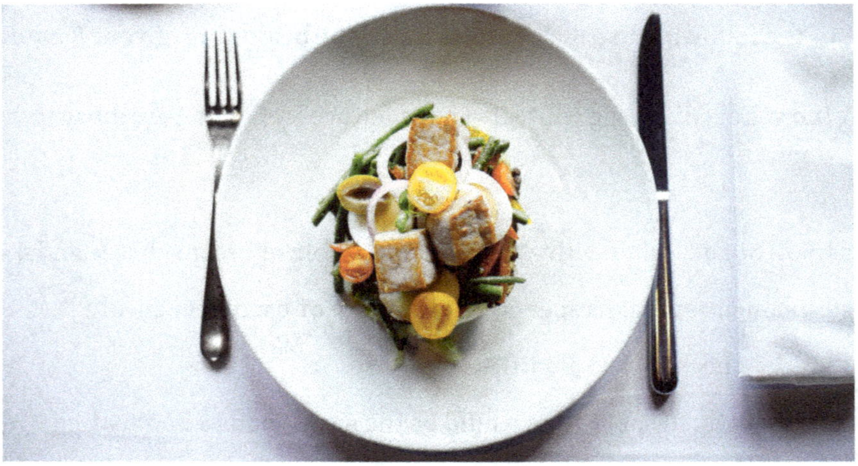

ReStart One Days 10 - 14

When you wake up, you'll enjoy a cup of hot water + 2 teaspoons of ACV (apple cider vinegar) and 1 teaspoon of lemon or lime juice.
 * If you substitute ACV capsules, make sure they contain "the mother".

Consume your liquid vitamins & minerals. You may consume by shooting or putting in water, coffee, or tea.

Greet the sun for 15 - 20 minutes with a bare face and without sunglasses. Ideally place your bare feet in the grass. Enjoy the dance of colors and the solitude.

Consume up to 2 cups (16 ounces/ 500 ml) of caffeinated beverages throughout the day. Consume black or with 1 teaspoon of high fat whipping cream, 1 teaspoon of unsweetened almond, coconut milk, or a carb free nut pod if desired, to each cup. Use liquid stevia as a sweetener.

Drink at least 72 ounces (2.25 liters) of water throughout the day.
At least 48 ounces (1.42 liters) of the fluid should be electrolyte enhanced. You can use Ultima, pink Himalayan salt, Smart water, etc.

You may consume an unlimited about of caffeine free herbal teas - either hot or cold.

DO NOT CONSUME any sugar-free sweet-tasting drinks, jello, popsicles or pudding. They will spike your blood sugar and prevent you from going into ketosis. However, you may freeze Ultima and make snow cones or popsicles.

Continue to choose one snack at the beginning of your 8 hour eating window and one at the end. In addition to the options above, you may now also choose from:

2 ounces of salmon or tuna mixed with 2 teaspoons avocado or full fat mayonnaise.

1 ounce of chicken or tofu mixed with 1 cup of napa lettuce and 2 teaspoons feta cheese. Top with apple cider vinegar, lemon juice or ½ teaspoon MCT oil. Personally, I like to mix the ACV & MCT oil. Spice to taste.

2 ounces of real lump crab meat (no imitation/ no fillers) heated in 2 teaspoons Kerry Gold Irish Butter. Spritz with lemon or lime.

During your one meal you will now choose 2 to 3 ounces of a dense protein source, such as beef, lamb, pork, or cod in addition to your veggie. You'll find dense protein more filling for a longer period of time. Consume at the time of your choosing during your 8 hour eating window.

REMEMBER TO EXERCISE

ALWAYS continue your medications and supplements. End your day by taking your probiotic just prior to going to bed. This will maximize the time it spends in your digestive tract. This is also the time to take your liquid calcium/magnesium in broth, herbal tea, Ultima or another liquid.

Drinking water is like washing out your insides. The water will cleanse the system, fill you up, decrease your caloric load and improve the function of all your tissues.
--Kevin R. Stone

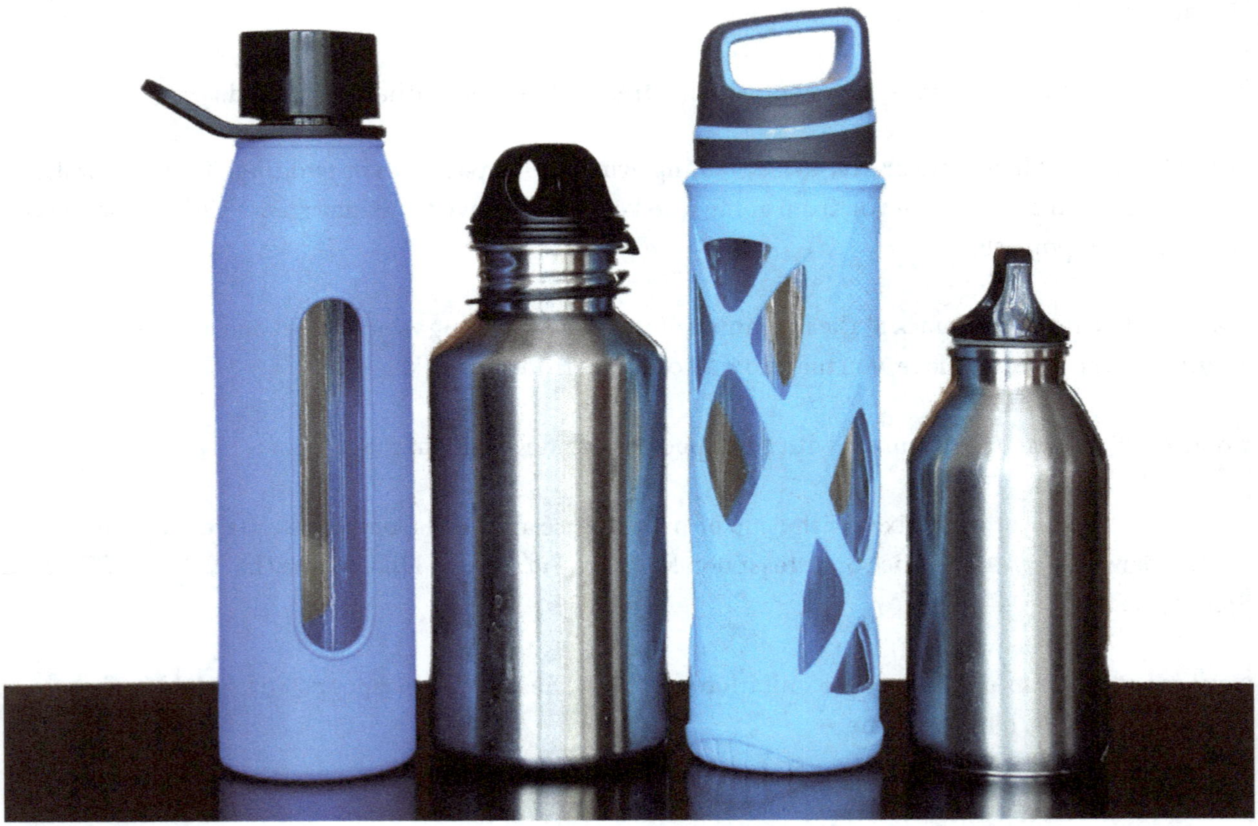

 Content provided in this book is of a general nature only and does not replace the information and advice provided by your own health care professionals. Always consult your own health care providers for specific personal health and medical advice.

Tips for Mindful Eating AFTER ReStart:

Be prepared. Keep bottles of water in your car and stevia in your purse. Carry beef jerky or cheese wafers in your purse.

Keep a feeding schedule and stick to it. For example, know that at 11 am you'll break your fast with an egg. At 1 pm you'll eat lunch and at 2:30 pm you'll have a snack. Between meals you'll have Ultima flavored water. In the morning you'll have a caffeinated beverage and again at 3 pm.

Your body will quickly adapt to the new feeding schedule and you'll experience less hunger between feedings. LOG EVERYTHING in your BariKeto app. Water, supplements, food, everything. Measure every morsel that passes your lips. We often underestimate how much we've consumed. Purchase a kitchen scale and use it daily.

Meal prep one day each weekend for the week ahead. By making most food in advance, you'll never be caught by surprise. Meal time during the week will be fast and easy. Simply heat up a prepared meal and steam veggies just before eating

Physical Hunger	vs.	Emotional Hunger
Comes on gradually & can be postponed		Comes on suddenly & feels urgent
Can be satisfied with any type of food		Causes specific cravings, Pizza, chocolate, ice-cream...
Once you're full you can stop eating		Eat more than you normally would. Feel uncomfortably full
Causes satisfaction, doesn't cause guilt		Leaves you feeling guilty & cross with yourself

5

PLAN

2

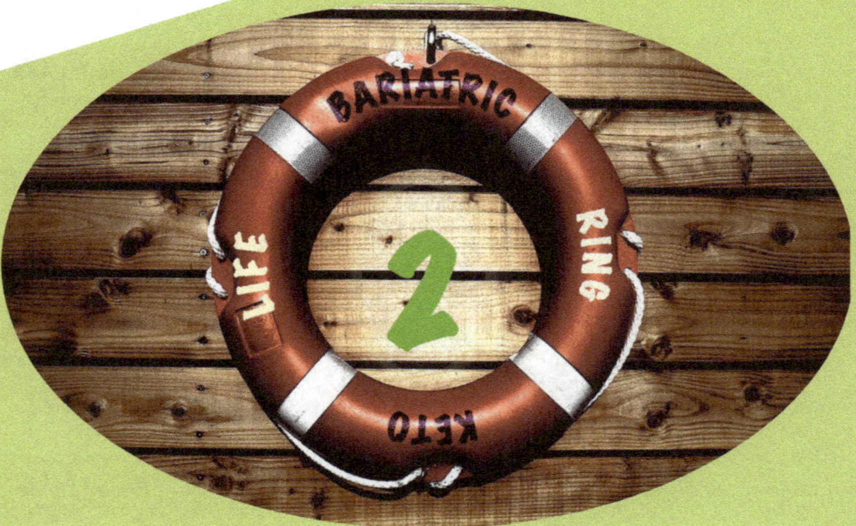

 Content provided in this book is of a general nature only and does not replace the information and advice provided by your own health care professionals. Always consult your own health care providers for specific personal health and medical advice.

If you're looking for a quick start to get your head in the game and the weight loss restarted, this is the plan for you. This option focuses on the gut-brain connection and how our minds and stomachs work in harmony to direct our decision making about food.

- Days 1 - 3: Consume nourishing liquids to feed your body while concentrating your energy on breaking old habits.
- Days 4 – 7: Concentrates on mindful eating and recognizing full signals.
- Days 8 – 10: Introduces new food options and ways to quiet your brain. Now is the time to purchase and schedule your 1:1 training so you'll have macros and be able to trnasition directly into our long term eating program.

- Days 8 - the rest of your life: Start with gentle exercises. Gradually increase at your own pace. Remember, exercise only accounts for 20% of weight loss and can actually drive you to consume more. Do it because it makes you feel more alive, lessens depression & anxiety, and helps move water out of your body so you get to experience those wonderful WOOSHes faster!

- Days 11 – 14: Encourages you to take stock of your ReStart Journey and reflect on what you've accomplished. Prepare to transition to the BariKeto method of eating.

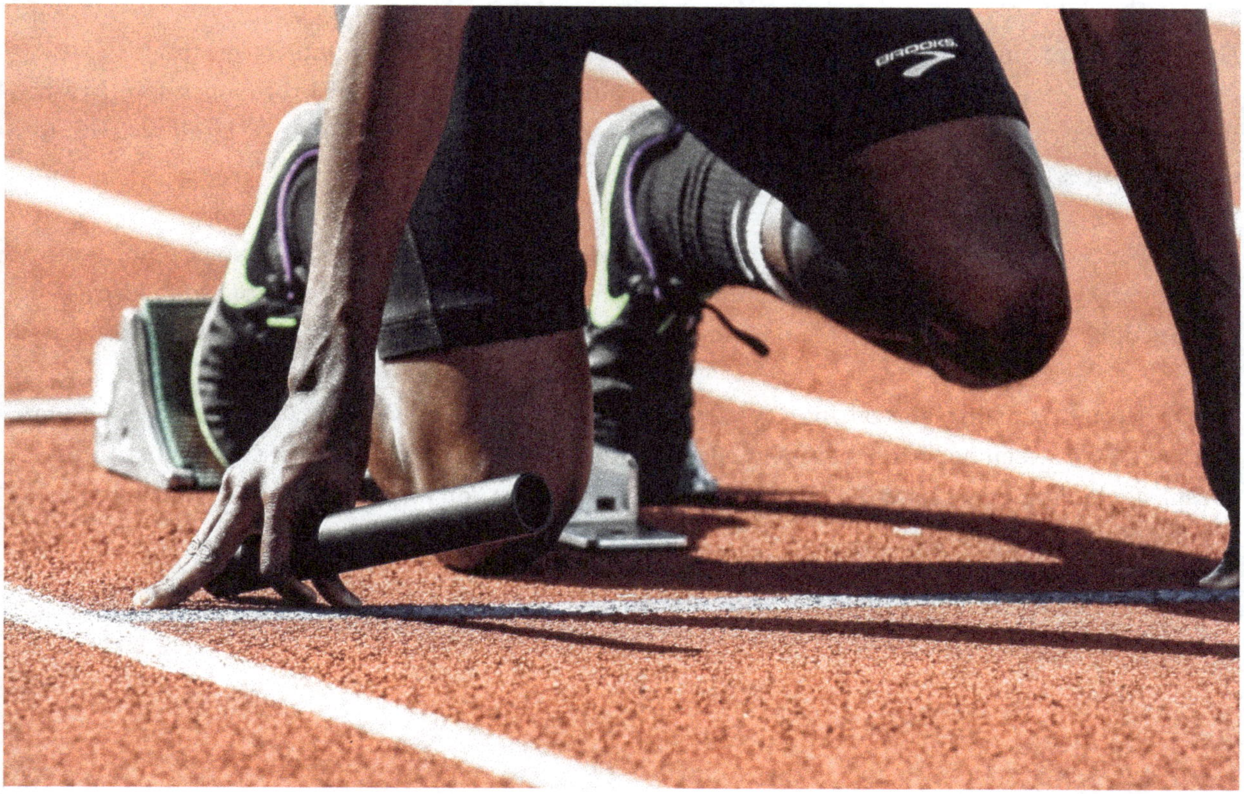

ReStart Plan Two – Days 1-3

Food intake will cease beginning the prior night no later than 10 pm. Schedule for a day you can concentrate on yourself with few distractions. Don't sabotage yourself by starting on a day with a high stress schedule. Make sure all food shopping has been accomplished prior to starting.

When you wake up, you'll enjoy a cup of hot water + 2 teaspoons of ACV (apple cider vinegar) and 1 teaspoon of lemon or lime juice.
* If you substitute ACV capsules, make sure they contain "the mother", it's the active ingredient.

Consume your liquid vitamins & minerals. You may consume by shooting or putting in water, coffee, or tea.

Greet the sun for 15 - 20 minutes with a bare face and without sunglasses. Ideally place your bare feet in the grass. Enjoy the dance of colors and the solitude.

Consume up to 2 cups (16 ounces/ 500 ml) of caffeinated beverages throughout the day. Consume black. You may add 1 teaspoon of unsweetened 1 teaspoon of unsweetened almond, coconut milk, or a carb free nut pod if desired, to each cup. Use liquid stevia as a sweetener.

Drink at least 72 ounces (2.25 liters) of water throughout the day. Broth counts in this total. Consume clear liquids only with all solids strained out. Broths such as bone broth, miso soup broth, pho broth, veggie soup broth, etc. Broth must be low sodium and contain no MSG. Limit yourself to 64 fluid ounces (8 cups) per day.

NOTE: For those with PCOS, thyroid or blood sugar issues, add ½ cup protein of choice and ½ cup non-starchy veggie of choice (total of 1 cup) to the 8 cups of broth on days 1 & 2. You won't lose as much weight, but it will keep you from washing out of the program due to fatigue or dizziness.

HINT: If you find plain water boring, try varying the temperature as well as size of ice cubes. You can also use stevia sweetened products ONLY, such as Ultima. No Splenda, sugar, or sugar substitutes except stevia. You may also infuse water with fruit or veggies. You may not, however, consume the veggies or squeeze them.

To enjoy good health, to bring true happiness to one's family, to bring peace to all, one must first discipline and control one's own mind. If a man can control his mind he can find the way to Enlightenment, and all wisdom and virtue will naturally come to him.

--Buddha

Prepare and drink one 8 ounce glass of your preferred flavor of e xogenous ketones, with or without caffeine. Do this during your "hump time" when you would normally want to grab a snack to keep going.

At least 48 ounces (1.42 liters) of the fluid should be electrolyte enhanced. You can use Ultima, pink Himalayan salt, Smart water, etc.
You may consume an unlimited about of caffeine free herbal teas - either hot or cold.

DO NOT CONSUME any sugar-free sweet-tasting drinks, jello, popsicles or pudding. They will spike your blood sugar and prevent you from going into ketosis. However snow cones or popsicles made from ultima are fine.

ALWAYS continue your medications and supplements. End your day by taking your probiotic just prior to going to bed. This will maximize the time it spends in your digestive tract. This is also the time to take your liquid calcium/magnesium in broth, herbal tea, Ultima or another liquid. Be prepared to spend a lot of time running to the toilet.

For me, first, it's finding quiet in my life - and I do that through yoga and meditation. It's also been a matter of changing the way I eat, because I think what we eat can inform who we are; food is a chemical and a drug to a certain extent.
--Mariel Hemingway

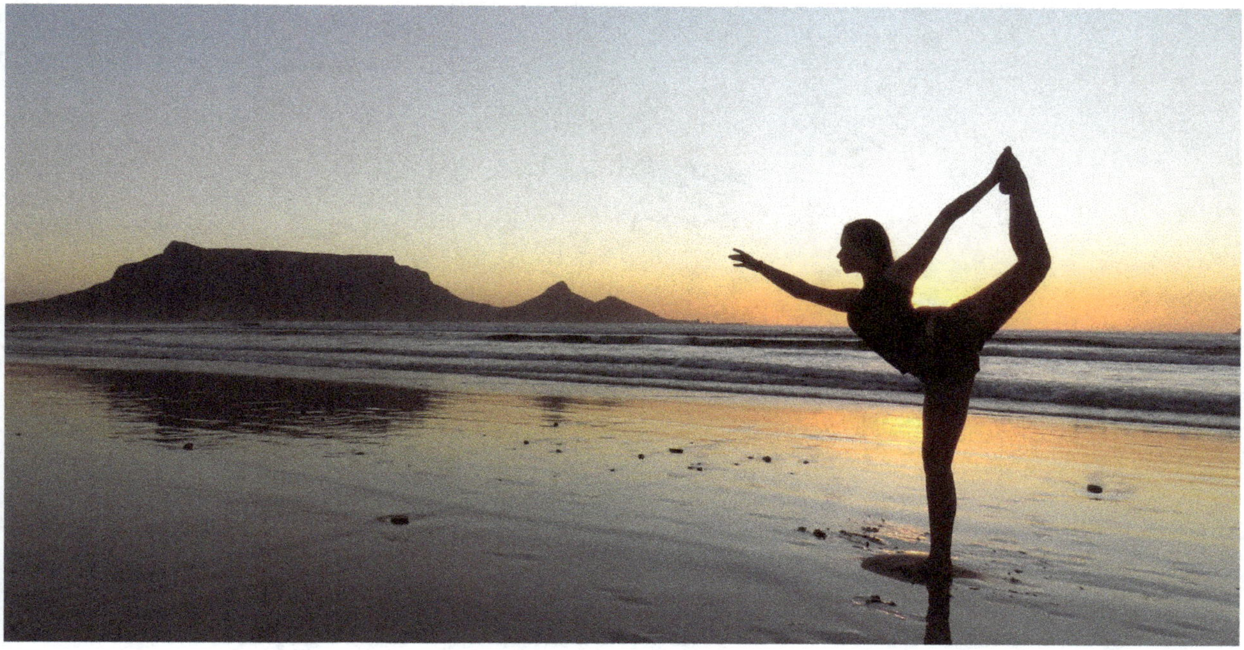

ReStart Plan Two Days 4 - 6

When you wake up, you'll enjoy a cup of hot water + 2 teaspoons of ACV (apple cider vinegar) and 1 teaspoon of lemon or lime juice.
* If you substitute ACV capsules, make sure they contain "the mother".

Consume your liquid vitamins & minerals. You may consume by shooting or putting in water, coffee, or tea.

Greet the sun for 15 - 20 minutes with a bare face and without sunglasses. Ideally place your bare feet in the grass. Enjoy the dance of colors and the solitude.

Consume up to 2 cups (16 ounces/ 500 ml) of caffeinated beverages throughout the day. Consume black, you may add 1 teaspoon of unsweetened almond, coconut milk, or a carb free nut pod if desired, to each cup. Use liquid stevia as a sweetener.

Continue to consume clear liquids with all solids strained out. Broths such as bone broth, miso soup broth, pho broth, veggie soup broth, etc. Broth must be low sodium and contain no MSG. Limit yourself to 32 fluid ounces (4 cups) per day.

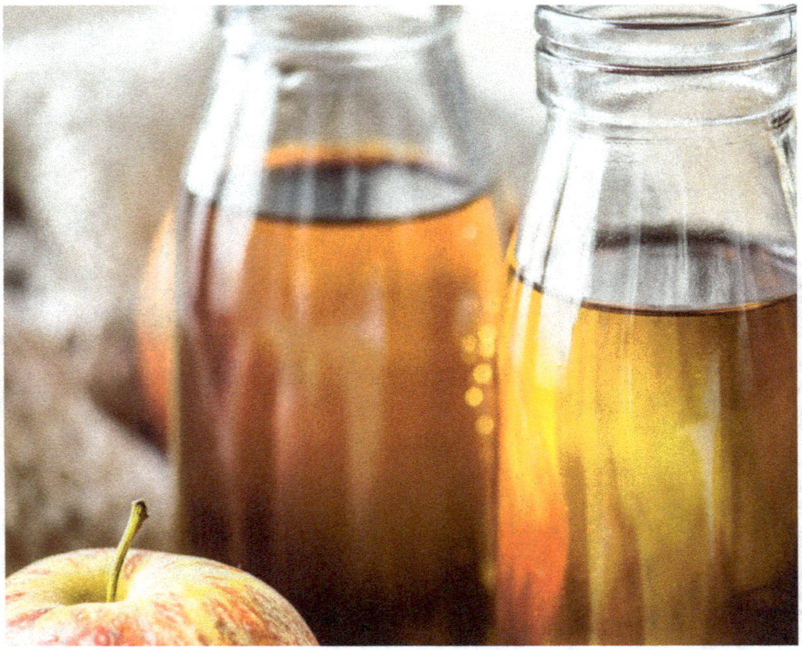

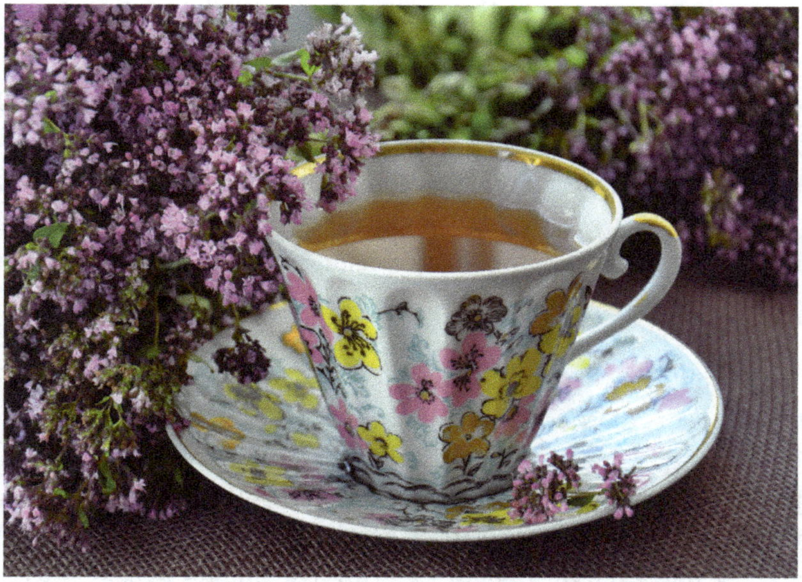

Tea makes everything better.
--Bindi Irwin

Drink at least 72 ounces (2.25 liters) of water throughout the day. Broth counts in this total. At least 48 ounces (1.42 liters) of the fluid should be electrolyte enhanced. You can use Ultima, pink Himalayan salt, Smart water, etc.

You may consume an unlimited about of caffeine free herbal teas - either hot or cold.

During days 4, 5 & 6 you will eat one meal each day. The meal will consist of 2 - 3 ounces of chicken or fish. Prepared grilled, poached or roasted. And ¼ - ½ cup of non-starchy veggies steamed or sautéed in olive oil or apple cider vinegar. You may add 1 teaspoon of Kerry Gold Irish Butter, if desired. Add pink Himalayan sea salt and/or pepper to taste. You may eat this meal at the time of your choosing, however, all of the meal must be consumed in one sitting.

DO NOT CONSUME any sugar-free sweet-tasting drinks, jello, popsicles or pudding. They will spike your blood sugar and prevent you from going into ketosis. However, you may freeze Ultima and make snow cones or popsicles.

ALWAYS continue your medications and supplements. End your day by taking your probiotic just prior to going to bed. This will maximize the time it spends in your digestive tract. This is also the time to take your liquid calcium/magnesium in broth, herbal tea, Ultima or another liquid.

ReStart Plan Two Days 7 - 9

When you wake up, you'll enjoy a cup of hot water + 2 teaspoons of ACV (apple cider vinegar) and 1 teaspoon of lemon or lime juice.
* If you substitute ACV capsules, make sure they contain "the mother".

Consume your liquid vitamins & minerals. You may consume by shooting or putting in water, coffee, or tea.

Greet the sun for 15 - 20 minutes with a bare face and without sunglasses. Ideally place your bare feet in the grass. Enjoy the dance of colors and the solitude.

Consume up to 2 cups (16 ounces/ 500 ml) of caffeinated beverages throughout the day. Consume black or with 1 teaspoon of high fat whipping cream. You may add 1 teaspoon of unsweetened almond, coconut milk, or a carb free nut pod if desired, to each cup. Use liquid stevia as a sweetener.

Continue to consume clear liquids with all solids strained out. Broths such as bone broth, miso soup broth, pho broth, veggie soup broth, etc. Broth must be low sodium and contain no MSG. Limit yourself to 16 fluid ounces (2 cups) per day.

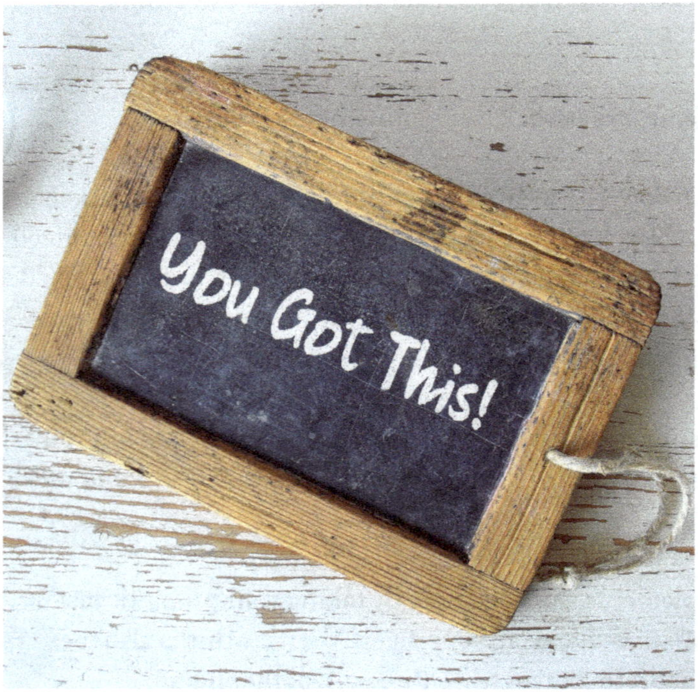

Drink at least 72 ounces (2.25 liters) of water throughout the day. Broth counts in this total.
At least 48 ounces (1.42 liters) of the fluid should be electrolyte enhanced. You can use Ultima, pink Himalayan salt, Smart water, etc.

You may consume an unlimited about of caffeine free herbal teas - either hot or cold.

DO NOT CONSUME any sugar-free sweet-tasting drinks, jello, popsicles or pudding. They will spike your blood sugar and prevent you from going into ketosis. However, you may freeze Ultima and make snow cones or popsicles.

Choose ONE one of the following to eat at what would be the beginning of your 8 hour eating window:

1 egg white ONLY (no yoke). Wrap egg white in a napa lettuce leaf (chinese cabbage) with 1 teaspoon of avocado mayo.

6 slices (4 ounces total) of cucumber with 2 tablespoons of feta or cream cheese and 6 almonds

(2) bacon-wrapped, steamed asparagus spears. Use one slice of bacon per spear.

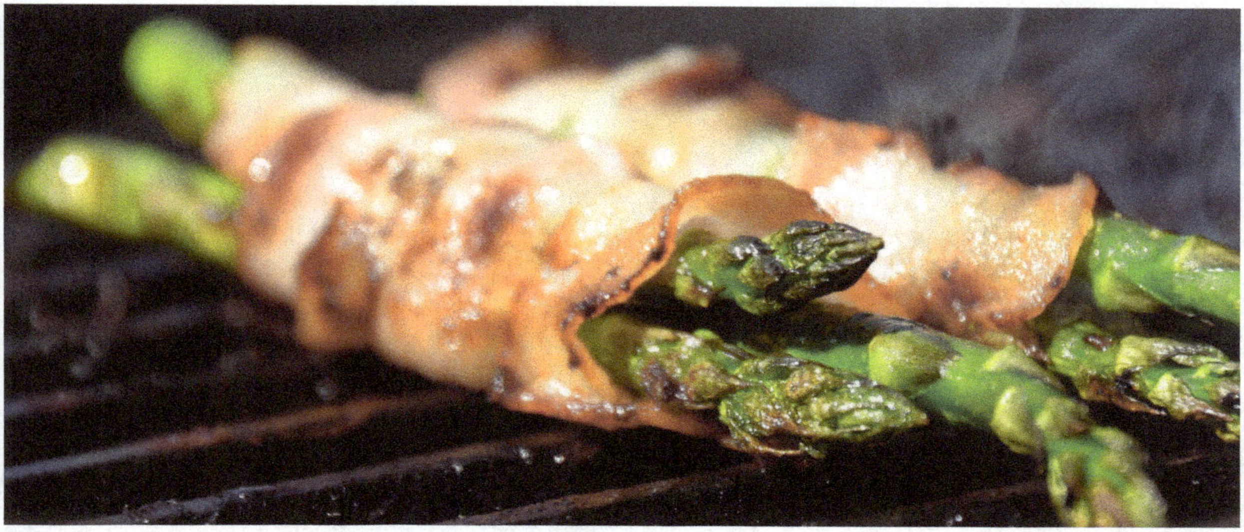

(3) one ounce of cheddar cheese (28.35 grams).

Choose ONE of the following to eat at what would be the end of your 8 hour eating window:

One large or two small dill pickles with one ounce of cheddar cheese (28.35 grams).

10 steamed or raw green string beans (not sugar snap) with 2 teaspoons feta or cream cheese

¼ cup blueberries or sliced strawberries in 1 tablespoon heavy whipping cream

1/2 ounce each of cooked chicken breast and oven roasted ham (not pre-cut sandwich meat) for a total of one ounce of meat.

In addition, consume your meal of 2 - 3 ounces of chicken or fish. Prepared grilled, poached or roasted. And ¼ - ½ cup of non-starchy veggies steamed or sautéed in olive oil or apple cider vinegar. You may add 1 teaspoon of Kerry Gold Irish Butter, if desired. Add pink Himalayan sea salt and/or pepper to taste. You may eat this meal at the time of your choosing, however, all of the meal must be consumed in one sitting.

ALWAYS continue your medications and supplements. End your day by taking your probiotic just prior to going to bed. This will maximize the time it spends in your digestive tract. This is also the time to take your liquid calcium/magnesium in broth, herbal tea, Ultima or another liquid.

A simple rule of thumb is to shop the periphery of the grocery store - that's where you'll find meat, fish, dairy, and vegetables. Choose high-quality protein such as healthy, grass-fed beef and lamb and organic chicken and pork, and eat them in moderation.

--Suzanne Somers

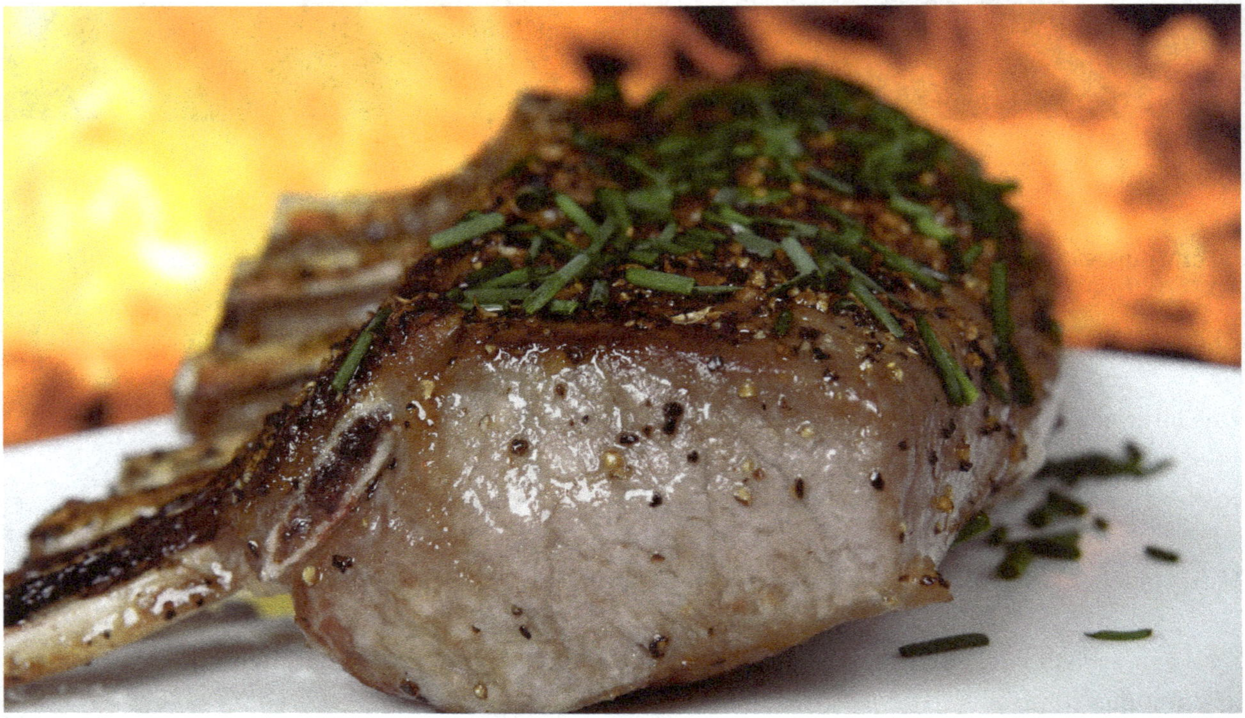

ReStart Two Days 10 - 14

When you wake up, you'll enjoy a cup of hot water + 2 teaspoons of ACV (apple cider vinegar) and 1 teaspoon of lemon or lime juice.
* If you substitute ACV capsules, make sure they contain "the mother".

Consume your liquid vitamins & minerals. You may consume by shooting or putting in water, coffee, or tea.

Greet the sun for 15 - 20 minutes with a bare face and without sunglasses. Ideally place your bare feet in the grass. Enjoy the dance of colors and the solitude.

Consume up to 2 cups (16 ounces/ 500 ml) of caffeinated beverages throughout the day. Consume black or with 1 teaspoon of high fat whipping cream, 1 teaspoon of unsweetened almond or coconut milk, or a nut pod, if desired, to each cup. Use liquid stevia as a sweetener.

Drink at least 72 ounces (2.25 liters) of water throughout the day. Broth counts in this total. At least 48 ounces (1.42 liters) of the fluid should be electrolyte enhanced. You can use Ultima, pink Himalayan salt, Smart water, etc.

You may consume an unlimited about of herbal teas - either hot or cold.

DO NOT CONSUME any sugar-free sweet-tasting drinks, jello, popsicles or pudding. They will spike your blood sugar and prevent you from going into ketosis. However, you may freeze Ultima and make snow cones or popsicles.

Continue to choose one snack at the beginning of your 8 hour eating window and one at the end. In addition to the options above, you may now also choose from:

2 ounces of salmon or tuna mixed with 2 teaspoons avocado or full fat mayonnaise.

1 ounce of chicken or tofu mixed with 1 cup of napa lettuce and 2 teaspoons feta cheese. Top with apple cider vinegar, lemon juice or ½ teaspoon MCT oil. Personally, I like to mix the ACV & MCT oil. Spice to taste.

2 ounces of real lump crab meat (no imitation/ no fillers) heated in 2 teaspoons Kerry Gold Irish Butter. Spritz with lemon or lime.
During your one meal you will now choose 2 to 3 ounces of a dense protein source, such as beef, lamb,

pork, or cod in addition to your veggie.. You'll find dense protein more filling for a longer period of time. Consume at the time of your choosing during your 8 hour eating window.

REMEMBER TO EXERCISE

ALWAYS continue your medications and supplements. End your day by taking your probiotic just prior to going to bed. This will maximize the time it spends in your digestive tract. This is also the time to take your liquid calcium/magnesium in broth, herbal tea, Ultima or another liquid.

Tips for Mindful Eating AFTER ReStart:

Be prepared. Keep bottles of water in your car and stevia in your purse. Carry beef jerky or cheese wafers in your purse.

Keep a feeding schedule and stick to it. For example, know that at 11 am you'll break your fast with an egg. At 1 pm you'll eat lunch and at 2:30 pm you'll have a snack. Between meals you'll have Ultima flavored water. In the morning you'll have a caffeinated beverage and again at 3 pm.
Your body will quickly adapt to the new feeding schedule and you'll experience less hunger between feedings. LOG EVERYTHING in your BariKeto app. Water, supplements, food, everything.

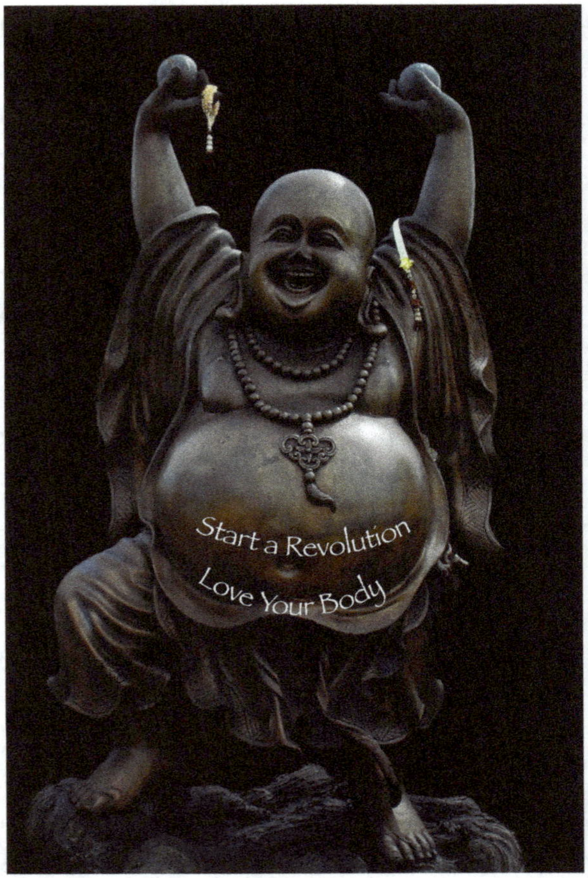

Measure every morsel that passes your lips. We often underestimate how much we've consumed. Purchase a kitchen scale and use it daily.
Meal prep one day each weekend for the week ahead. By making most food in advance, you'll never be caught by surprise. Meal time during the week will be fast and easy. Simply heat up a prepared meal and steam veggies just before eating

KEEP EXERCISING AND MOVING

 Content provided in this book is of a general nature only and does not replace the information and advice provided by your own health care professionals. Always consult your own health care providers for specific personal health and medical advice.

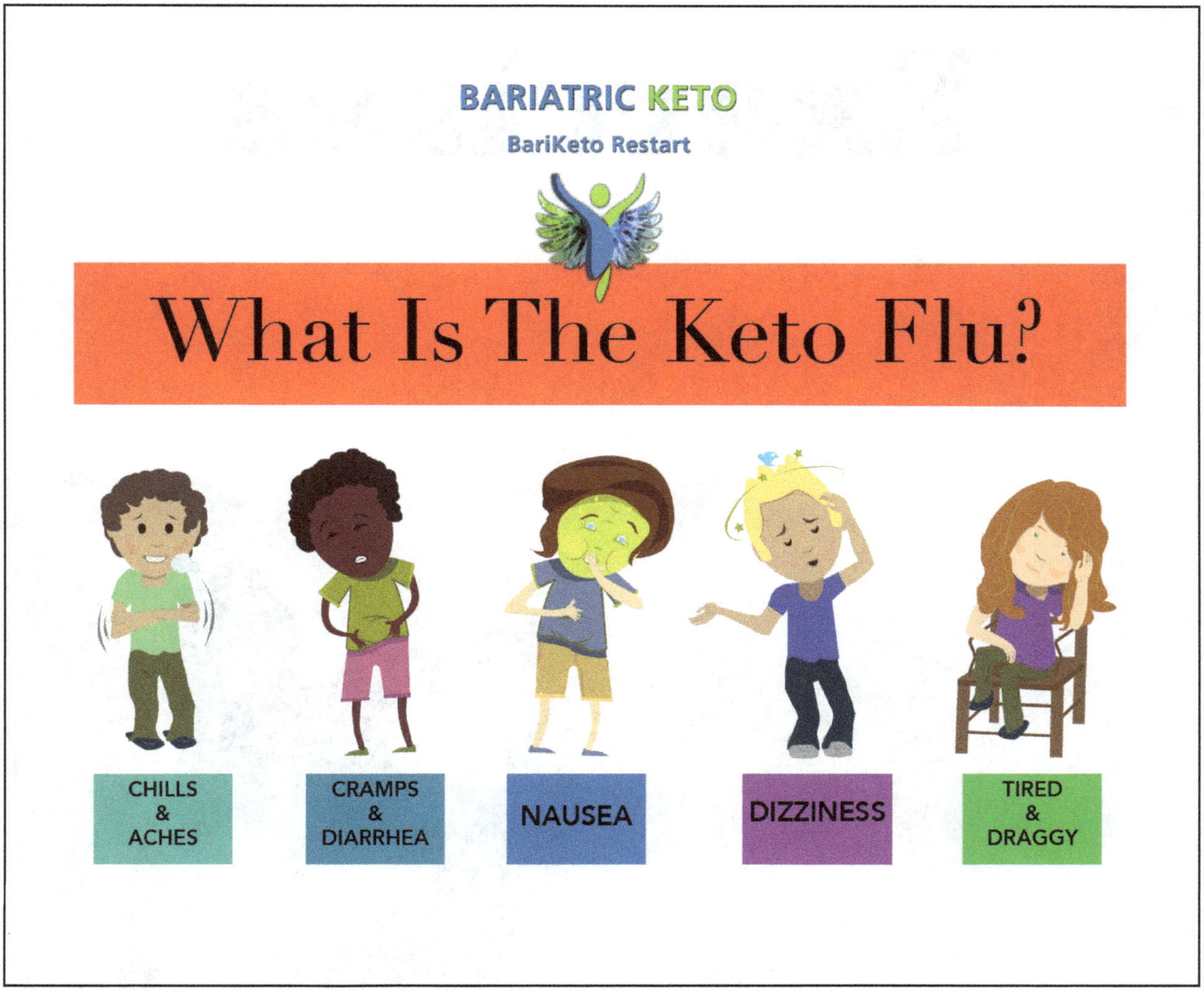
BARIATRIC KETO
BariKeto Restart
What Is The Keto Flu?
CHILLS & ACHES
CRAMPS & DIARRHEA
NAUSEA
DIZZINESS
TIRED & DRAGGY

6

Mindfulness Exercises

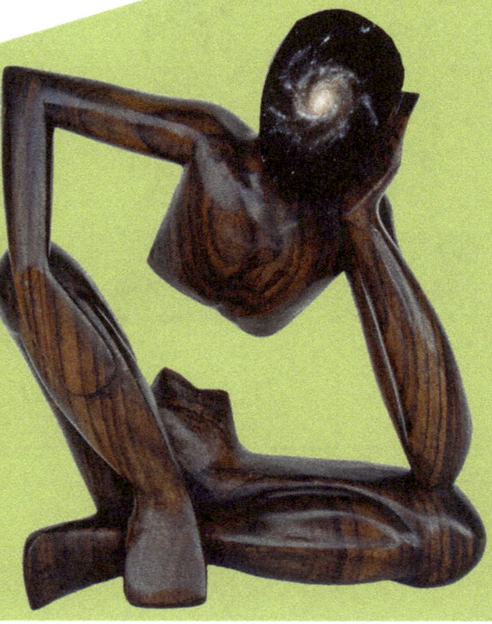

Mindfulness exercises will address what drives you to want food. This is a journey of self discovery and love. I personally think it's one of the most important journeys I've ever undertaken. Each time I go through ReStart this part is always new and illuminating. The outside world is nonstop fast paced. Don't let it infect your inside world of calm acceptance.

Twice each day I'm going to ask you to carve out time for yourself from your day. The times you choose are up to you. I find first thing in the morning and last thing at night are most beneficial to my energy levels, sleep patterns and inner calm

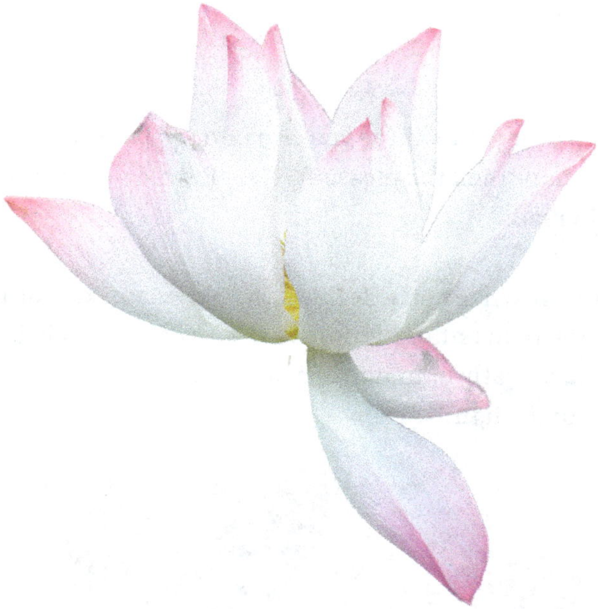

Eating from memories. We associate food with family, warmth and love. Our mothers and grandmothers taught us in the kitchen and over family meals. Food was loaded with family togetherness and created special memories.

Strive today to break that cycle for yourself and those you love.

- Sit around a campfire singing songs and telling stories rather than eating s'mores.
- Take a pickle and water to the movie theater.
- Go to the park to play and have fun without the picnic.
- Celebrate a birthday by volunteering rather than eating cake.
- Log into our support groups and helps someone going through something you just experienced.

MINDFULNESS DAY 1:

Did you know taking a long 30 minute soak in a warm bath burns as many calories as walking 20 minutes?

What you'll need:

- Epsom salts (¼ cup - ½ cup)
- A good book
- Essential oil (whatever scent you prefer)
- At least 40 minutes of quiet time
- Rich body lotion

Take time to feel the water creep over your skin as you slip into the bathtub. Settle back as you feel the warm water envelop your limbs and smell the pleasant oils. Revel in the solitude and quiet of your bathroom. When ready, start to read.

Have a thick, thirsty towel available when you exit the bath. Blot your skin rather than rubbing briskly. Immediately apply lotion to maximize absorption. Cover your body in slow, swirling strokes with the lotion. Then exit the warm bathroom into cool air to close your skin's pores. Ideally, you'll be able to slip into bed for an incredible night's sleep.

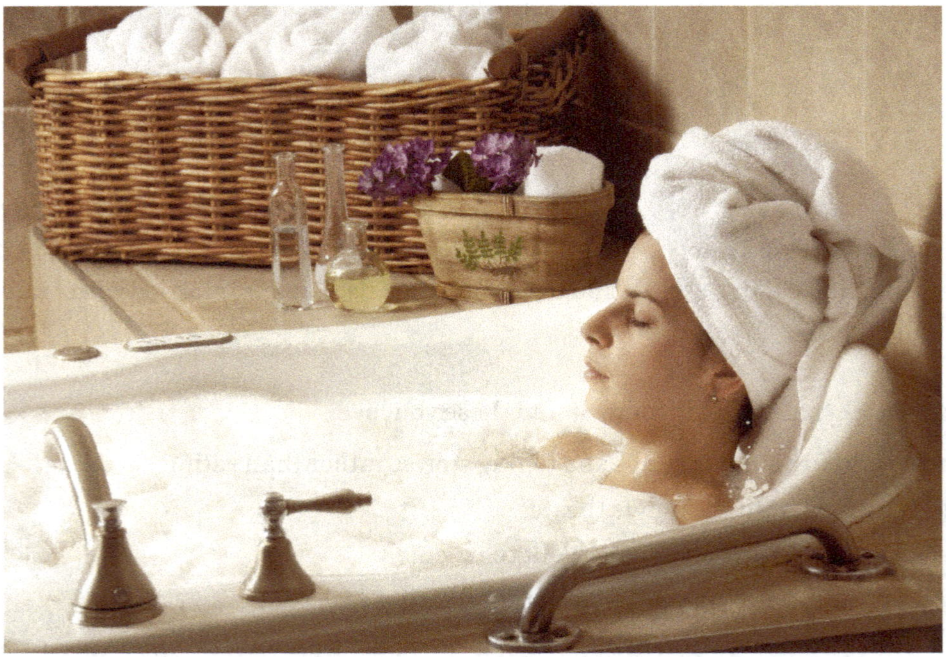

 Content provided in this book is of a general nature only and does not replace the information and advice provided by your own health care professionals. Always consult your own health care providers for specific personal health and medical advice.

MINDFULNESS DAYS 2 - 9

Prepare your meal and place it on the table. Stand next to your chair and notice the color and texture of the food in front of you. Settle gently into your chair. Inhale the aroma of the food. Do the smells remind you of anything? Take a small bite of the food. Put your utensil down as you study the food in your mouth. Feel the fat coat your tongue. Taste the spices on the top of your tongue. How does the taste differ as it travels to the back of your tongue? Chew each bite 20 times prior to swallowing. Pick up your utensil and repeat the process. Do not force yourself to finish the portion of food. Stop as soon as you feel satiated or you receive your full signal. Know that being a member of the "clean plate club" never got you anywhere but obese.

MINDFULNESS DAYS 2B - 9B

Clear a space for quiet sitting. It can be in a garden, a room, or a closet. Wherever you'll be able to sit for 20 minutes without being disturbed.

What you'll need:

- A timer or your phone
- Music for meditation - select ahead and download
- A towel or pillow
- A candle, incense, or object of special meaning

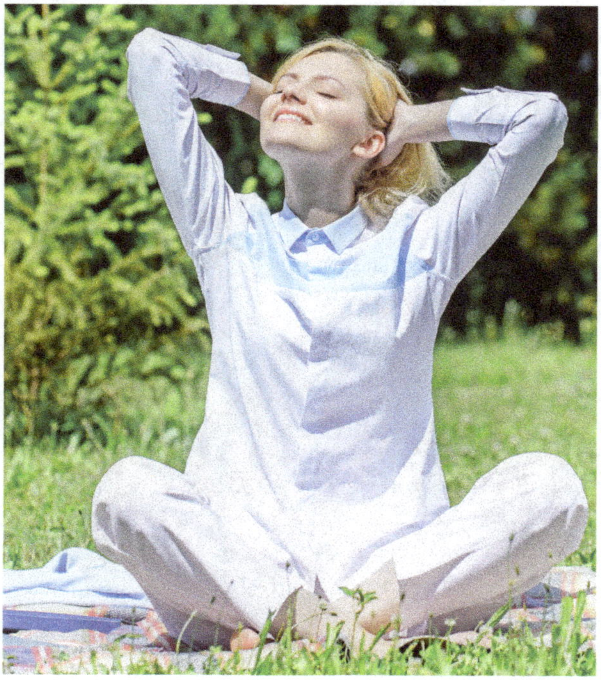

If using your phone, turn off the ringer. Set the timer for 10 minutes and settle into the seated area you prepared. Using correct posture, turn on the soft music and close your eyes. Your goal is to follow your breathing. Note the chest's rise and fall. Feel your stomach expand with each breath in and then contract as your breath is released. If your thoughts stray, bring them back into focus. Rest your hands comfortably in your lap. Breath in contentment and peace. Breath out restless anxiety. You will hold this position until the timer rings. Try not to squirm and continue to bring your thoughts back to your breathing. Breath in light and breath out darkness. Over the next week gradually increase your mindfulness time from 10 - 20 minutes

MINDFULNESS DAYS 10 - 14

Begin your day with easy stretching for 10 minutes. Next, if the weather is nice, move outside for 10 minutes of walking. Go at the pace that best suits you. If the weather threatens, move briskly inside for 10 minutes. Don't think ahead to what your day will contain. Keep your mind focused on your body and why you are making this journey.

MINDFULNESS DAYS 10B - 14B

Take the calm centeredness you've begun to feel during your alone time on the road with you. When you find yourself in a stressful situation, remove yourself by saying, "I'll get back to you in just a minute". Few things in life truly are emergencies that must be acted on immediately. Lower your stress level by knowing how to distinguish between them. Remove yourself physically from the stressor and breathe slow breaths. Breathe in peace. Breathe out stress. Know you can deal with this situation and have faith in your ability.

End your day with a warm soak in Epsom Salts followed by lotion. Slip beneath clean sheets knowing you did your best today. Tomorrow holds the promise of weight loss, increased energy and clarity of purpose.

EXTRA CREDIT EXERCISE:

Buy yourself the garment you picture yourself wearing at goal weight. Hang it on your closet door and imagine how you'll look and feel wearing it. Know the struggle is worth it - you are worth it! Think of all the people you give to daily. Know you can't fill a cup from an empty pitcher. Resolve to refill your pitcher each night so you have compassion to give each day.

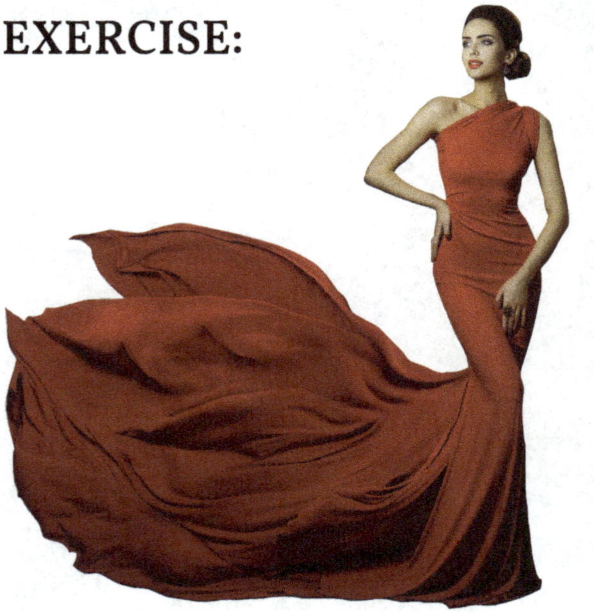

Next Steps:

If you have not already done so, it's time to purchase your 1:1 training and transition to full time Bariatric Keto eating. The simplest way is using your assigned macros on our menu app. It will tell you what to eat in order to achieve your goal weight.
Purchase at www.BariatricKeto.com

There's no reason to eat off plan when our Bariatric Keto menu app does all the counting for you. Simply purchase the shopping list of ingredients at your grocery store & prepare the food as shown. When you eat to plan, logging food is easy – and the custom macros you receive during training ensure you'll lose the excess weight in a healthy intelligent manner.

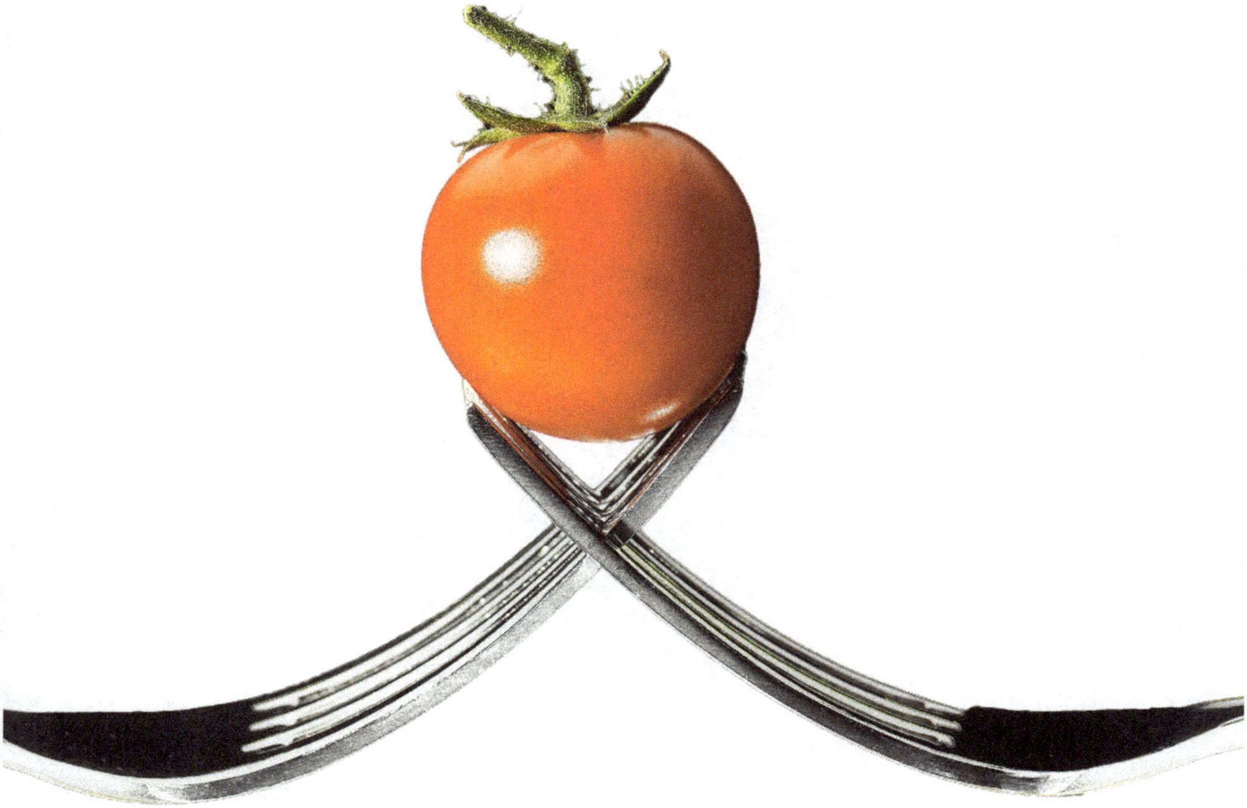

Too little is it considered, while we gaze on aristocratic beauty, how much good food, soft lying, warm wrapping, ease of mind, have to do with the attractions which command our admiration.

--Samuel Lover

7

APPENDICES

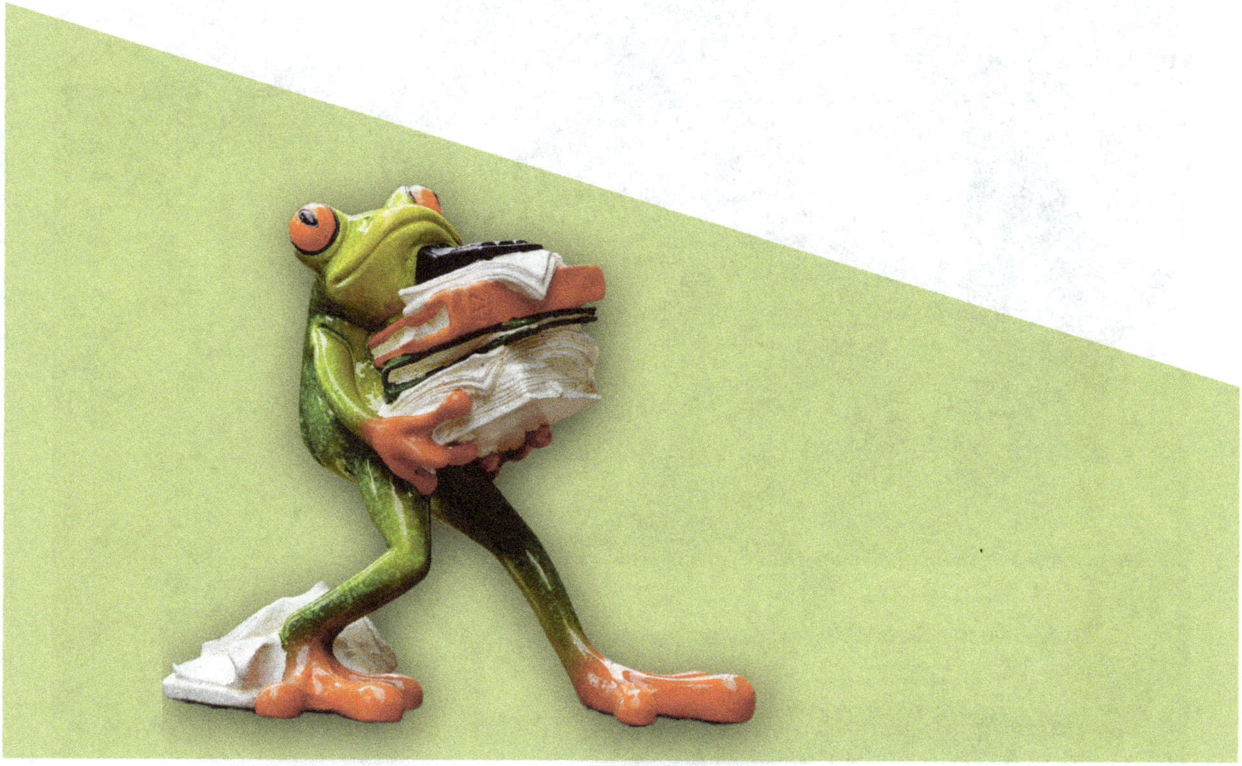

Appendix A-Recipes

This is not an exhaustive list of recipes, nor are you required to use these recipes if you don't desire. They are supplied for your convenience. Feel free to use other sources such as Pinterest for Keto-friendly recipes that you will need during your ReStart.

Cooking is one of the strongest ceremonies for life. When recipes are put together, the kitchen is a chemical laboratory involving air, fire, water and the earth. This is what gives value to humans and elevates their spiritual qualities. If you take a frozen box and stick it in the microwave, you become connected to the factory.
--Laura Esquivel

https://www.pinterest.com/bariatricketo/?eq=bariatric%20keto&etslf=23251

https://www.facebook.com/groups/423596911345242/

https://www.youtube.com/channel/UCm4ZYoxQ346ABLLoYH-YxaA/videos

@BariatricK

For more great recipe ideas visit:
bariatricketo.com

BONE BROTH

Start with good quality bones/chicken frames, preferably organic and hormone-free.
Add 1/4-1/2 cup vinegar (depending on how large a batch your making)
Add any vegetables as you'd like, and water to cover. Because of their extremely high nutritional content, be sure to add some dark leafy greens to the mix.

Let this sit for 30 minutes to an hour. This allows the vinegar to leech vital nutrients out of the bones.

Bring to a boil and remove any scum that appears on the surface.
Continue to simmer anywhere from 4-24 hours. The longer the simmer, the more nutrients will be drawn out of the bones.

When done, measure your 1 cup serving size into mason jars and store in the fridge for when you need them.

To make a vegetable broth: Make the same way, simply omit the bones.

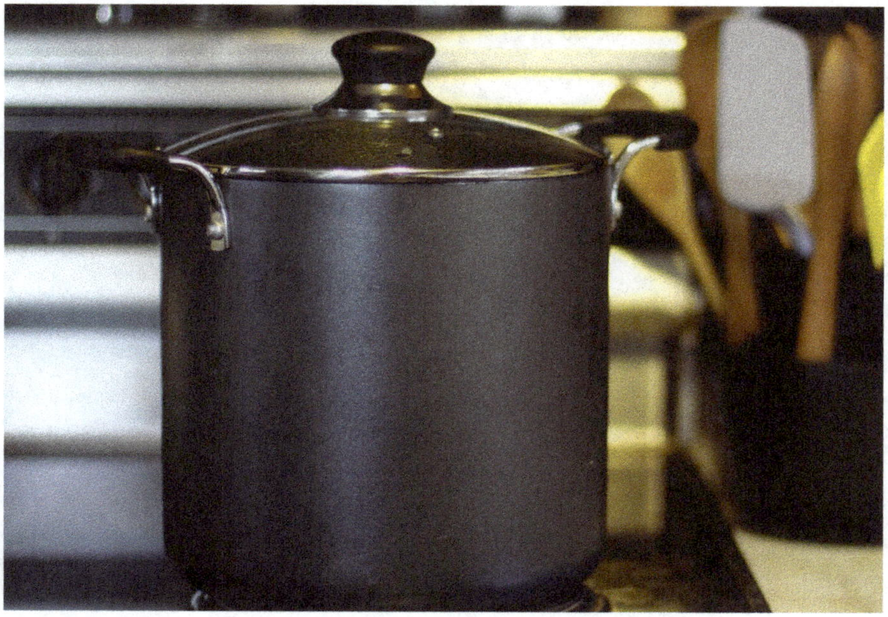

EGG DROP SOUP

(Great for chunky broth)

INGREDIENTS

1 1/2 cups chicken/bone broth
1 tablespoon bacon fat or butter
2 large eggs
1 teaspoon chili garlic paste

METHOD

Put a pan on the stove and turn it to medium-high heat. Add the chicken broth and bacon fat or butter to the pan. Bring it to a boil, add the chili garlic paste and stir. Turn off stove. Beat the eggs and pour into the steaming broth. Stir and let sit for approximately 30 seconds. Serve and enjoy!

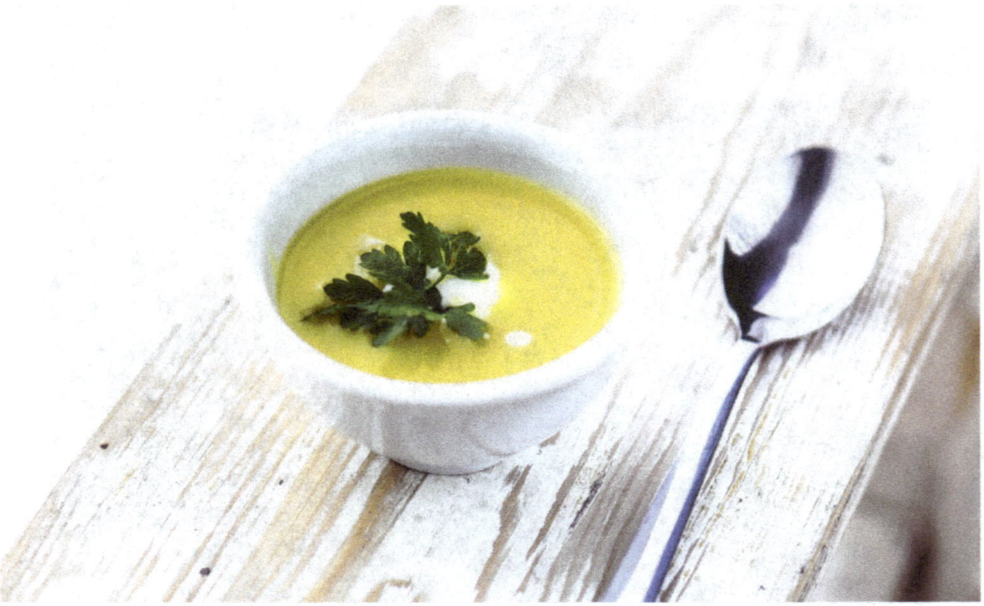

CABBAGE SOUP RECIPE

INGREDIENTS

2 large onions
2 green peppers
1 bunch of celery
1 head of cabbage
2 tablespoons coconut oil
6–8 cups of water or bone broth

METHOD

Chop all vegetables into cubes.
In a large stock pot, sauté onions in the coconut oil.
Then add the remaining vegetables and cover with water or bone broth and other seasonings, if desired.
Bring to a boil, then reduce to medium heat. Let simmer until vegetables are tender, about 30–45 minutes.
You may season the soup with salt, pepper, hot sauce, herbs or spices.
STRAIN FOR BROTH

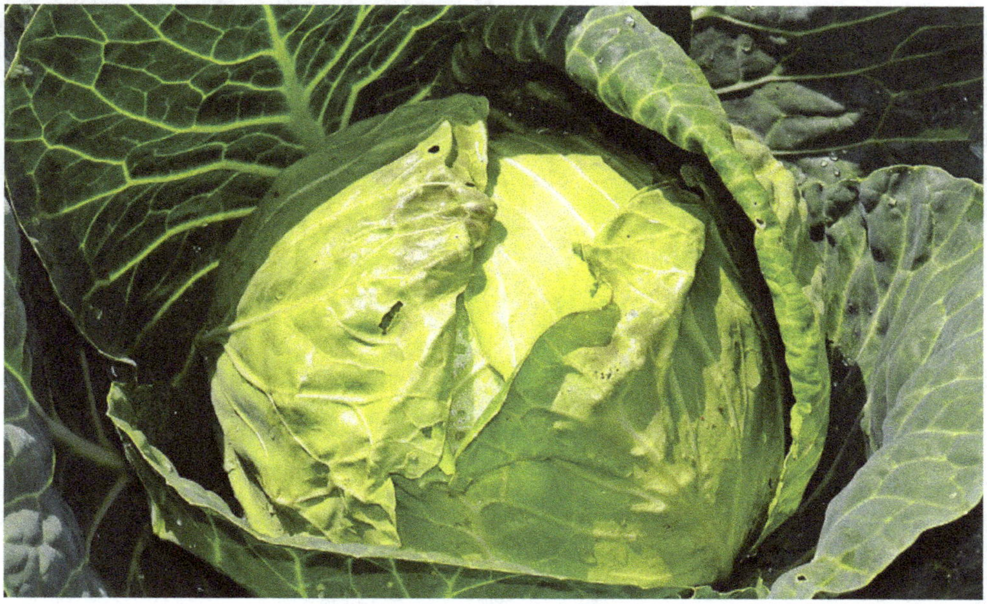

KETO BEEF JERKY

INGREDIENTS

2 pounds choice, raw Beef, Flank, or Steak, lean only, trimmed to 0" fat
2 tablespoons Liquid Smoke
1 teaspoon paprika
1 teaspoon table salt
1/4 cup Worcestershire Sauce
2 tablespoons Soy Sauce - Kikkoman 'Lite'
1 teaspoon garlic powder
1 teaspoon onion powder
1 teaspoon black pepper

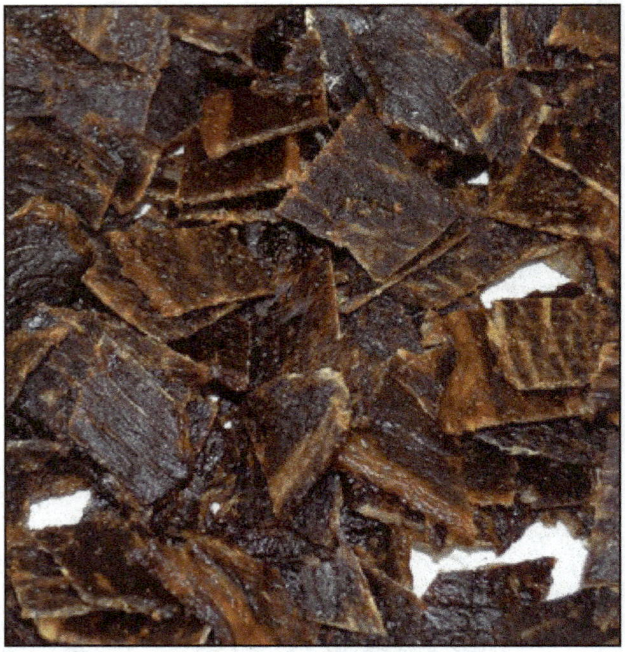

METHOD

Cut steak into thin strips.
Place in a large zip lock bag.
Add all other ingredients to the bag and mix thoroughly.
Refrigerate overnight.
Place beef strips in a dehydrator and dry to your liking (at least 4 hours).
Keep refrigerated.

Makes 160 servings.

THAI COCONUT GINGER SOUP

4 standard servings or 8 post-WLS servings

INGREDIENTS

2 cups coconut milk
2 cups reduced-sodium chicken broth
6 quarter-size slices fresh ginger
1 stalk fresh lemongrass, cut in 1-in pieces or the zest of ½ lemon
1 pound boneless, skinless chicken breast or thighs, cut into small bite-sized chunks
1 cup sliced mushrooms
1 tablespoon fresh lime juice
1 teaspoon liquid Stevia
1 teaspoon Sriracha
1/4 cup fresh basil leaves
1/4 cup fresh cilantro
2 tablespoons olive or coconut oil

METHOD

In a skillet, heat the oil on medium heat and add the chicken. Cook thoroughly.
While the chicken is cooking, add the remaining ingredients to a medium saucepan and simmer until hot but not boiling.
Add the chicken and simmer for an additional five minutes.

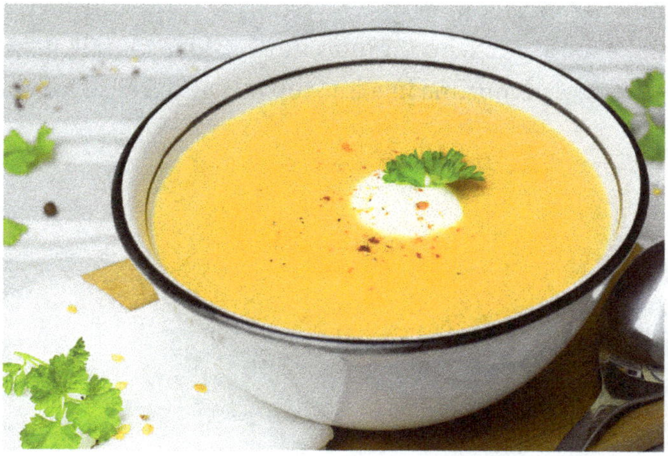

SAVORY CHEESE & TOFU MUFFINS

INGREDIENTS

6 medium eggs
2 tablespoons oil - olive or any nut oil.
10 g. Tuscan Seasoning
30 g. Parmesan cheese, grated
1 medium leek, sliced
15 g. minced garlic
Chicken stock cubes
large strips of bacon
150 g. cheddar cheese,grated
500 g. firm organic tofu, crumbled
1 container (247.5 g) chopped spinach (frozen)
Salt and pepper
3 tbsp. psyllium husk

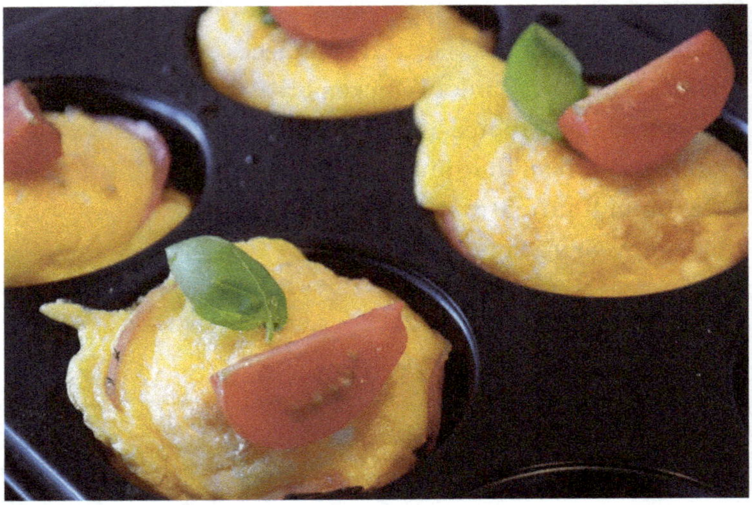

METHOD

Preheat your oven to 180°C/360°F
Add everything to a bowl, crumbling the tofu, chopping the bacon, adding the eggs and mixing together.
Use cupcake trays and muffin liners, divide the mix into 24 (approx. 1 heaped tablebspoon of wet mix per muffin liner)
Bake for approx. 20 minutes until golden and firm. Let cool and enjoy
Put cooled muffins in a zip-top bag and freeze for convenience

SMALL MEAL IDEAS

Small meals *contain 1½-2 oz. of dense protein any of the following:*
Beef, chicken, turkey, fish, pork, lamb, game meat, shrimp or tofu.
Your ***main meal*** *contains 2-3 oz. (no more) of dense protein.*

Butter and garlic sautéed asparagus with poached egg and parmesan cheese.

Cook asparagus and top with egg and parmesan

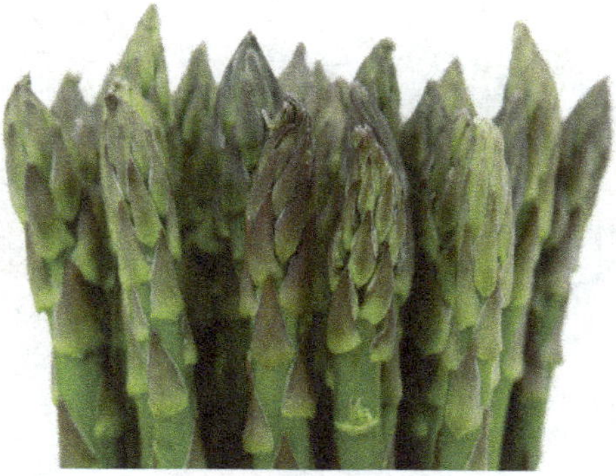

Grilled bacon wrapped cheesy asparagus

Sauté asparagus until tender, remove from heat.
Lay out 3 pieces of bacon and lay 2 asparagus spears on each.
Add a sprinkle of grated cheddar and parmesan cheese, roll up and place back in frying pan until bacon is crisp.

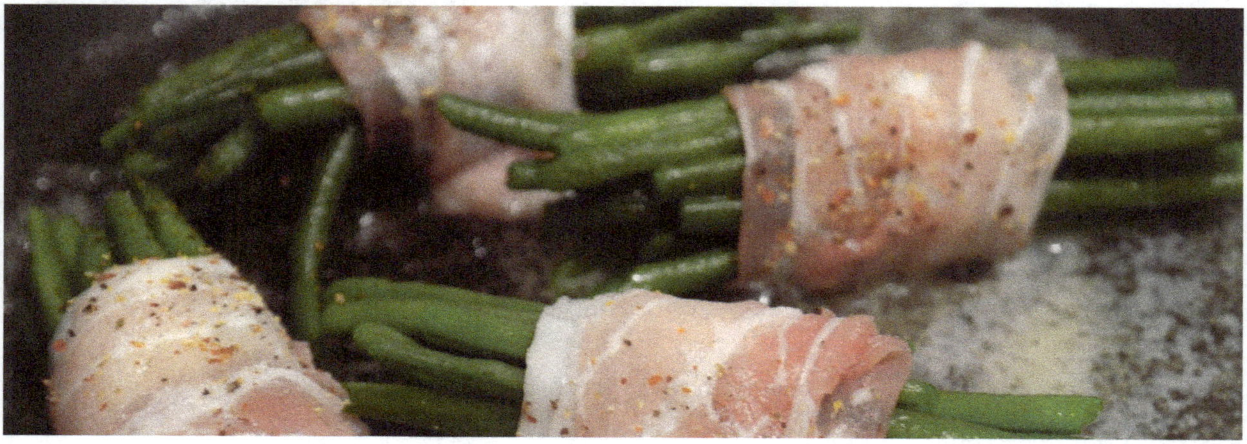

GRILLED SALMON & AVOCADO SALAD

1/2 cup of green salad leaves, 2oz. of grilled salmon
1/4 avocado sliced
Dress with a vinaigrette made of 1 Tbsp. Apple Cider Vinegar,
1 tablespoon Olive oil,
1 tsp. Lemon juice, salt and pepper

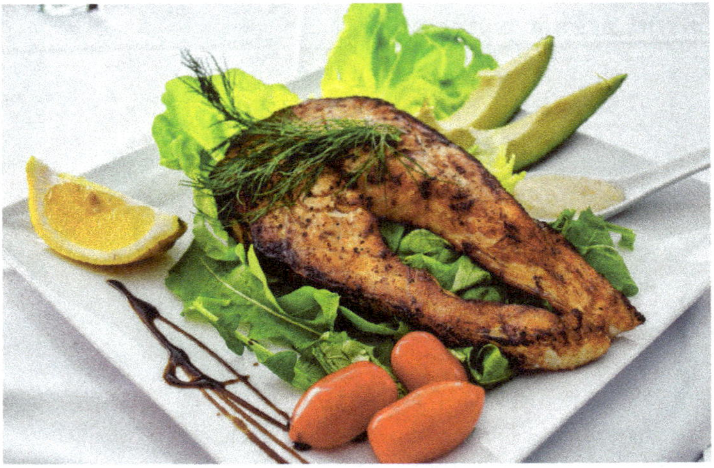

AVOCADO DEVILED EGGS

Boil 4-6 medium sized eggs.
Allow to cool and then peel.
Slice eggs in half and gently remove the yolks, emptying into a bowl.
Add to the yolks, 1/2 an Avocado, 1 tablespoon white vinegar, 1 teaspoon curry powder, salt and pepper, 1 teaspoon lemon juice and mix until smooth.
Using a spoon or piping bag, refill the hollows with the mix.
Place the halves in a container with a lid and store in the refrigerator.
Eat 2 halves for your snack, or together with some green salad leaves for your meal.

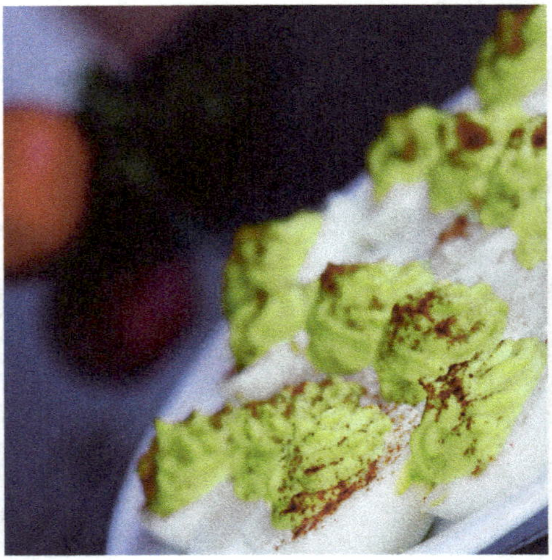

 Content provided in this book is of a general nature only and does not replace the information and advice provided by your own health care professionals. Always consult your own health care providers for specific personal health and medical advice.

SALADS

You can't seem to go wrong with salad and you are only limited by your imagination. Only use bok choy, napa lettuce, or spinach. You can try chicken and Persian feta on baby spinach with radish. Make a Caesar salad (without croutons) and add almonds. Try a warm Thai beef salad, exchanging noodles for thin zucchini ribbons, use fresh mint, cilantro/coriander and parsley together with baby spinach and dressed with sesame oil, chili and fish sauce.

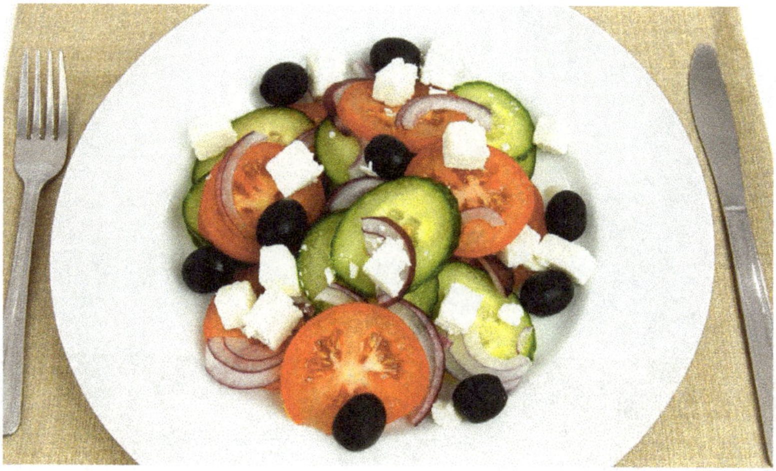

HERBAL ICED TEA

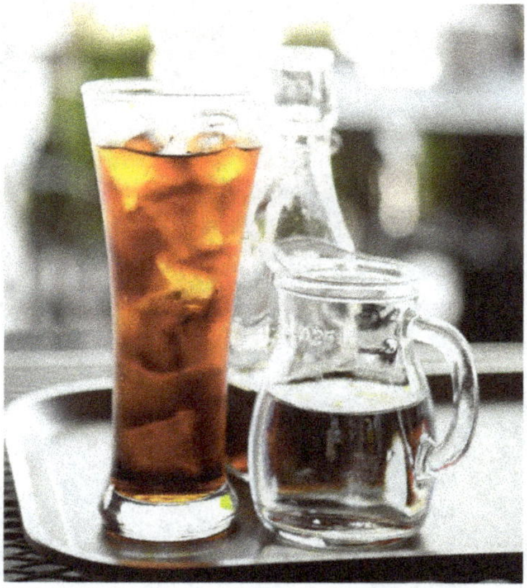

For a cool refreshing drink, why not make iced herbal tea? Steep 4-6 bags/servings of your favorite herbal tea in 2 cups of boiling water and let sit for 1-2 hours.
When cool, mix with 4 cups cold water and 1-2 tablespoons of lemon or lime juice.
You may like to slice the lemons and/or a 1 inch piece of ginger sliced finely; steep them in the boiling water for a zesty treat.

BARIATRIC KETO: WHAT TO EXPECT

Member Reviews

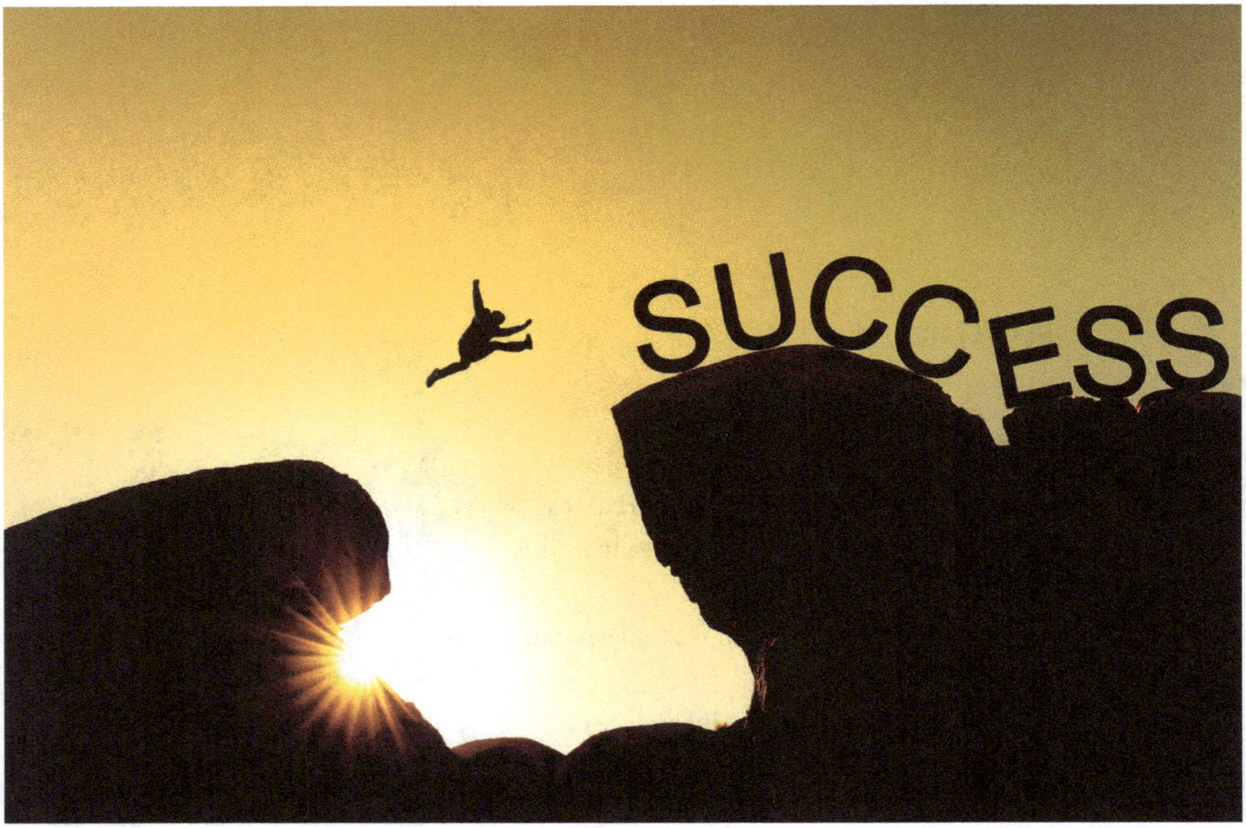

 Content provided in this book is of a general nature only and does not replace the information and advice provided by your own health care professionals. Always consult your own health care providers for specific personal health and medical advice.

You are reaching the end of your ReStart, and you are getting ready to transition into the Bariatric Keto pro gram. You have cleared your body and your mind and have set yourself up to move forward. We are proud of you and welcome you to join the multitudes of weight loss surgery patients who achieve wonderful results through the program. Here's what some of them have to say about Bariatric Keto:

"So, this happened this morning. I'M IN THE 240'S!!"
-Angie

"I have lost about 5 or 6 lbs. in a week and a half. Rock on!"
-Monica

"It's Wednesday Weigh Day. Down 3 pounds in one week. 178"
-Sheryl

"Just had my one on one. 1:1 OMG soooo helpful! Thanks!!"
-Jodi

"...stalled for 3.5 [months]... started Keto and now the last 20-25 lbs. are starting to melt off"
-Michelle

"14 day ReStart done! I am down 20.8 pounds! I feel fantastic. It was so worth sticking with it!"
-Terri

"I have been doing really well... following the plan and losing nearly a pound a day... the plan works if you work it."
-Cathleen

"My 1:1 mentor session was wonderful. I feel like I have a much better understanding of the Keto plan. I have the information in writing to review as needed. I highly recommend you have your one on one if you need Information and encouragement"

-Pamela

"I love Keto. Finally found what works for me. Thank you! 40lbs down in 3 months!!"

-Sherry

For the first time in three years I feel hope. I'm down 16.8 pounds. For any ladies on the fence, this is a great program and worth every head hunger.

-Amber

"I appreciate what you've done for me. I lost 3 pounds since our 1:1. I'm really sticking to this. Thanks again!!"

-Wanda

"Thanks so much for the 1:1 last night, so much great information!"

-Cindy

"Just finished ReStart #1!!!! Lost 15 pounds!!!!! The secret? Change your mindset by focusing on YOU and doing the homework!!!

-Sarah

REFERENCES

Because we like to back up our claims with hard core research

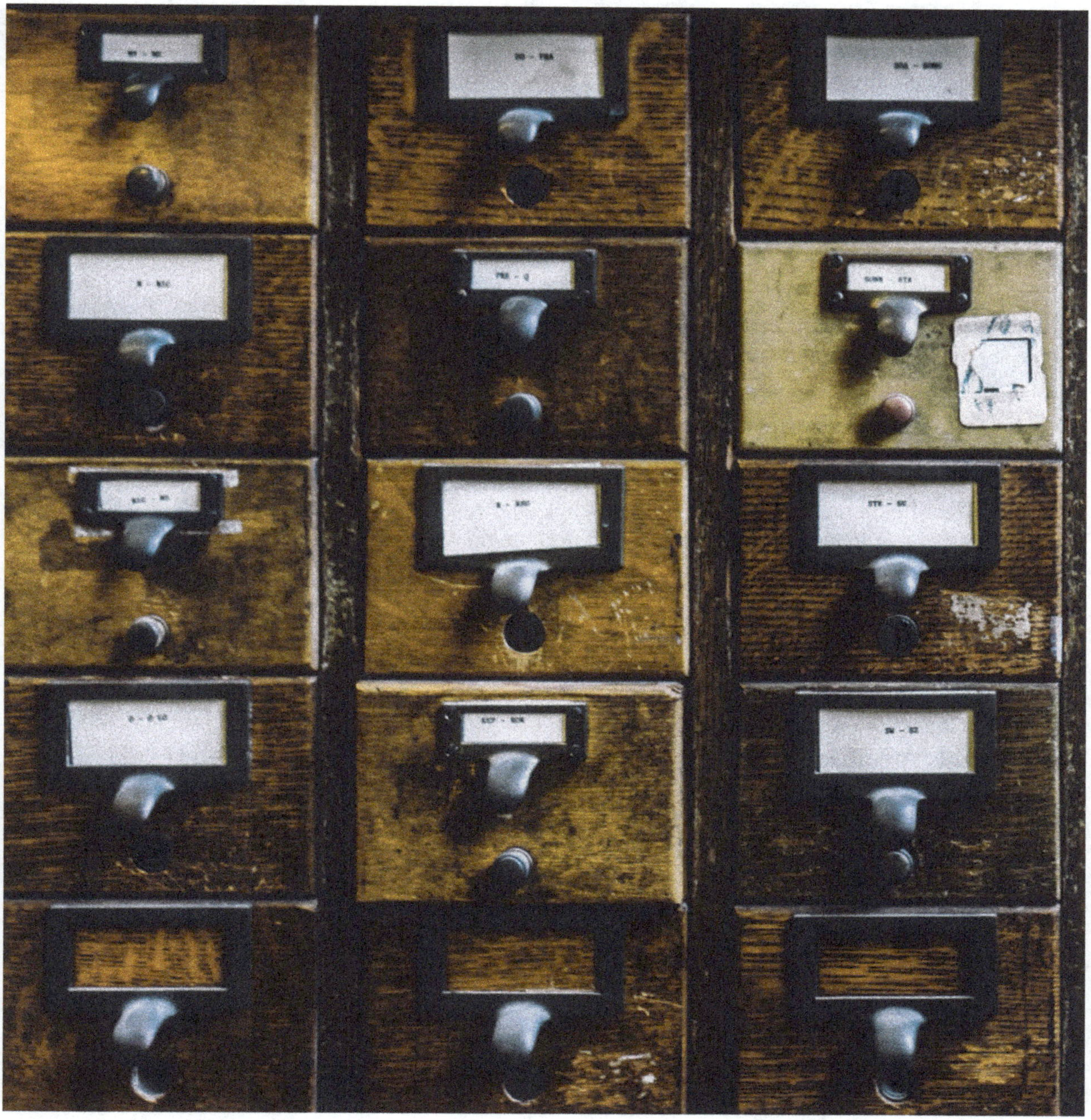

Baur, L. A., Twigg, S. M., & Magnusson, R. S. (2012). A modern epidemic: Expert perspectives on obesity and diabetes. Sydney: Sydney University Press.

Adler, E., Dhruva, A., Moran, P. J., Daubenmier, J., Acree, M., Epel, E. S., … Hecht, F. M. (2017). Impact of a Mindfulness-Based Weight-Loss Intervention on Sleep Quality Among Adults with Obesity: Data from the SHINE Randomized Controlled Trial. Journal of Alternative & Complementary Medicine, 23(3), 188–195.

Aniys, A. (2017) Alkaline plant based diet: reversing disease and saving the planet with an alkaline plant based diet. North Charleston, South Carolina: CreateSpace Independent Publishing.
Ahmad, J., Kohkan, G., Yusufi, F., Zafar, N., & Hasan, S. (2017). Impact of one-on-one education session on diabetes management and HbA1c in type 2 diabetes. Indian Journal of Endocrinology & Metabolism, 21, 54.

Altman, D. (2014). The Mindfulness Toolbox : 50 Practical Tips, Tools & Handouts for Anxiety, Depression, Stress & Pain. Eau Claire, Wisconsin: PESI Publishing & Media.

Aranow C. (2011). Vitamin D and the immune system. Journal of investigative medicine: the official publication of the American Federation for Clinical Research, 59(6), 881-6.

Arora, S. K., & McFarlane, S. I. (2005). The case for low carbohydrate diets in diabetes management. Nutr Metab (Lond), 2. https://www.ncbi.nlm.nih.gov/pubmed/16018812

Asadollahi, T., Khakpour, S., Ahmadi, F., Seyedeh, L., Tahami, Matoo, S., & Bermas, H. (2015). Effectiveness of mindfulness training and dietary regime on weight loss in obese people. Journal of Medicine & Life, 8, 114–124.

Basu, A., Rhone, M., & Lyons, T. J. (2010). Berries: emerging impact on cardiovascular health. Nutrition Reviews, 68 (3), 168–77. https://www. ncbi.nlm.nih.gov/pmc/articles/PMC3068482/

Beattie, J., Crozier, A., & Duthie, G. (2005). Potential Health Benefits of Berries. Current Nutrition & Food Science, 1 (1), 71–86. http://www. eurekaselect.com/79477/article

Boden, G., Sargrad, K., Homko, C., Mozzoli, M., & Stein, T. P. (2005). Effect of a low-carbohydrate diet on appetite, blood glucose levels, and insulin resistance in obese patients with type 2 diabetes. https://www.ncbi.nlm.nih.gov/pubmed/15767618

Boyer, J., & Liu, R. H. (2004). Apple phytochemicals and their health benefits. Nutrition Journal, 3, 5. https://nutritionj.biomedcentral.com/articles/10.1186/1475-2891-3-5

Brand-Miller, J., Hayne, S., Petocz, P., & Colagiuri, S. (2003). Low–Glycemic Index Diets in the Management of Diabetes: A meta-analysis of randomized controlled trials. Diabetes Care, 26(8), 2261–2267. https://www.ncbi.nlm.nih.gov/ pubmed/12882846Brand-Miller, Jennie, Ambler, & Geoffrey. (2012).

Braun, L., & Cohen, M. (2011). Herbs & Natural Supplements- An Evidence Based Guide (3rd ed.). Churchill Livingstone Elsevier.

Bray GA, Smith SR, Dejonge L, de Souza R, Rood J, Champagne CM, … Rood. (2012). Effect of diet composition on energy expenditure during weight loss: the POUNDS LOST Study. International Journal of Obesity, 36(3), 448–455.

Brenner, D. M., Moeller, M. J., Chey, W. D., & Schoenfeld, P.S. (2009). The Utility of Probiotics in the Treatment of Irritable Bowel Syndrome: A Systematic Review. The American Journal of Gastroenterology, 104(4), 1033–1049. https://www.ncbi.nlm.nih.gov/ pubmed/19277023

Brewer, J. A., Ruf, A., Beccia, A. L., Essien, G. I., Finn, L. M., Lutterveld, R. V., & Mason, A. E. (2018). Can Mindfulness Address Maladaptive Eating Behaviors? Why Traditional Diet Plans Fail and How New Mechanistic Insights May Lead to Novel Interventions. Frontiers in Psychology,9. doi:10.3389/ fpsyg.2018.01418

Brown, J. E. (2011). Nutrition through the Life Cycle (Fourth). Belmont, California: Cengage Learning.

Brown-Riggs, C. (2018). Bariatric Surgery's Role in Managing Type 2: Learn about the different procedures available and strategies for counseling patients. Today's Dietitian, 20(8), 44–47.

Bures, J., Cyrany, J., Kohoutova, D., Förstl, M., Rejchrt, S., Kvetina, J., … Kopacova, M. (2010). Small intestinal bacterial overgrowth syndrome. World Journal of Gastroenterology, 16(24), 2978–90. https://www.ncbi.nlm.nih.gov/pubmed/20572300

Caldwell, K. L., Baime, M. J., & Wolever, R. Q. (2012). Mindfulness Based Approaches to Obesity and Weight Loss Maintenance. Journal of Mental Health Counseling, 34(3), 269.

Caramoci, A., Mitoiu, B., Pop, M., Mazilu, V., Vasilescu, M., Ionescu, A. M., & Eugenia, R. (2016). Is intermittent fasting a scientifically-based dietary method? Sports Medicine Journal / Medicina Sportivâ, 12(2), 2747–2755.

Carroll, K. K. (2014). Current perspectives on nutrition and health. Montréal: Published for the Royal Society of Canada by McGill-Queens University Press.

de Carvalho, A., Jr., Turato, E. R., Chaim, E. A., & Magdaleno, R., Jr. (2014). Weight regain among women after metabolic and bariatric surgery: A qualitative study in Brazil. Trends in Psychiatry and Psychotherapy, 36(3), 140–146.

Chambers, M. (2015). Bariatric Surgery : Prevalence, Complications and Impact on Quality of Life. New York: Nova Science Publishers, Inc.

Chaput, J.-P., Després, J.-P., Bouchard, C., & Tremblay, A. (2012). Longer sleep duration associates with lower adiposity gain in adult short sleepers. International Journal of Obesity, 36(5), 752–756. https://www.ncbi.nlm.nih.gov/pubmed/21654631

Complementary and alternative medicine: Breakthroughs in research and practice. (2019). Hershey, Pennsylvania: IGI Global.

Denke, M. A. (2001). Metabolic effects of high-protein, low- carbohydrate diets. Am J Cardiol, 88. https://www.ncbi.nlm.nih.gov/pubmed/11423059

Eilender, E. (2016). Nutrition throughout the lifecycle. New York: Momentum Press.

Fung, T. T., Rimm, E. B., Spiegelman, D., Rifai, N., Tofler, G. H., Willett, W. C., & Hu, F. B. (2001). Association between dietary patterns and plasma biomarkers of obesity and cardiovascular disease risk. The American Journal of Clinical Nutrition, 73(1), 61–67. Retrieved from http://ajcn.nutrition.org/content/73/1/61.abstract

Gannon, M. C., & Nuttall, F. Q. (2004). Effect of a high-protein, low-carbohydrate diet on blood glucose control in people with type 2 diabetes. Diabetes, 53. https://www.ncbi.nlm.nih.gov/pubmed/15331548

Gasbarrini, A., Lauritano, E. C., Gabrielli, M., Scarpellini, E., Lupascu, A., Ojetti, V., & Gasbarrini, G. (2007). Small Intestinal Bacterial Overgrowth: Diagnosis and Treatment. Digestive Diseases, 25(3), 237–240. https://www.ncbi.nlm.nih.gov/pubmed/17827947

Gasche, C., Berstad, A., Befrits, R., Beglinger, C., Dignass, A., Erichsen, K. Van Assche, G. (2007). Guidelines on the diagnosis and management of iron deficiency and anemia in inflammatory bowel diseases. Inflammatory Bowel Diseases, 13(12), 1545–1553. https://www.ncbi.nlm.nih.gov/pubmed/17985376

German, J. B., & Dillard, C. J. (2006). Composition, structure and absorption of milk lipids: a source of energy, fat-soluble nutrients and bioactive molecules. Critical Review in Food Science and Nutrition, 46(1), 57–92. https://www.ncbi.nlm.nih.gov/pubmed/16403683

Goldman, B. (2018). Researchers aim to harness microbes in our intestines to cure what ails us : the doctor is in your gut. Stanford Medicine, 34(3), 26–45.

Gottschall, E. (2004). Breaking the Vicious Cycle - Intestinal Health Through Diet (Rev. ed.). Ontario, Canada: Kirk ton Press Ltd.

Gropper, S. S., & Smith, J. L. (2013). Advanced Nutrition and Human Metabolism (6th ed.). Wadsworth: Cengage Learning.

Gutierrez-Repiso, C., Soriguer, F., Rubio-Martn, E., Esteva de Antonio, I., Ruiz de Adana, M. S., Almaraz, M. C., … Rojo- Martinez, G. (2014). Night-time sleep duration and the incidence of obesity and type 2 diabetes. Findings from the prospective Pizarra study. Sleep Medicine, 15(11), 1398–1404. https://www.ncbi.nlm.nih.gov/pubmed/25262361

 Content provided in this book is of a general nature only and does not replace the information and advice provided by your own health care professionals. Always consult your own health care providers for specific personal health and medical advice.

Hall RM, Parry Strong A, & Krebs JD. (2016). Importance of low carbohydrate diets in diabetes management. Nutrition and Dietary Supplements, Vol 2016, Issue 1, Pp 9-19 (2016), (Issue 1), 9.

Hartwig, M. (2016). FOOD FREEDOM FOREVER: Letting go of bad habits, guilt and anxiety around food. Boston: Houghton Mifflin Harcourt.

HL. Cook, R., J. O, D. N., E. Donges, C., M. Parker, H., Lun Cheng, H., S. Steinbeck, K., ... T. O, C. H. (2017). Relationship between Obesity and Cognitive Function in Young Women: The Food, Mood and Mind Study. Journal of Obesity, 2017(1).

Horne, B. D., Muhlestein, J. B., & Anderson, J. L. (2015). Health effects of intermittent fasting: hormesis or harm? A systematic review. The American Journal of Clinical Nutrition, 102(2), 464–70.

Hu, F. B. (2003). Plant-based foods and prevention of cardiovascular disease: an overview. The American Journal of Clinical Nutrition, 78(3), 544S–551S.

Jeukendrup, A., & Gleeson, M. (2010). Sports Nutrition: An Introduction to Energy Production and Performance (Second). Champaign, IL: Human Kinetics.

Juranić, Z., & Žižak, Ž. (2005). Biological activities of berries: From antioxidant capacity to anti-cancer effects. BioFactors, 23(4), 207–211.

Kesten, D., & Scherwitz, L. (2015). Whole-person Integrative Eating: A Program for Treating Overeating, Overweight, and Obesity. Integrative Medicine: A Clinician's Journal, 14(5), 42–50.

Kerr, M., & Cafasso, J. (2017). Malabsorption Syndrome. Retrieved August 10, 2017, from https://www.healthline.com/health/malabsorption

Kerry, R. G., Patra, J. K., Gouda, S., Yooheon Park, Han-Seung Shin, & Das, G. (2018). Benefaction of probiotics for human health: A review. Journal of Food & Drug Analysis, 26(4), 927–939.

Klein, S., Sheard, N. F., Pi-Sunyer, S., Daly, A., Wylie-Rosett, J., Kulkarni, K., & Clark, N. G. (2004). Weight management through lifestyle modification for the prevention and management of type 2 diabetes: rationale and strategies. A statement of the American Diabetes Association, the North American Association for the Study of Obesity, and the American So. Am J Clin Nutr, 80. https://www.ncbi.nlm.nih.gov/pubmed/15277143

Kreykes, A., Choxi, H., & Rothberg, A. (2017). Post-bariatric surgery patients: Your role in their long-term care. Journal of Family Practice, 66(6), 356–363.

Kossoff, E. H., & Hartman, A. L. (2012). Ketogenic diets: new advances for metabolism-based therapies. Current Opinion In Neurology, 25(2), 173–178. https://www. ncbi.nlm.nih.gov/pubmed/22322415

Liu, S. (2002). Intake of Refined Carbohydrates and Whole Grain Foods in Relation to Risk of Type 2 Diabetes Mellitus and Coronary Heart Disease. Journal of the American College of Nutrition, 21(4), 298–306. Retrieved from https://www.ncbi.nlm.nih.gov/ pubmed/12166526

Lin, S. C., & Cheifetz, A. S. (2018). The Use of Complementary and Alternative Medicine in Patients With Inflammatory Bowel Disease. Gastroenterology & Hepatology, 14(7), 415–425.

Magee, L., & Hale, L. (2012). Longitudinal associations between sleep duration and subsequent weight gain: A systematic review. Sleep Medicine Reviews, 16(3), 231– 241. https://www.ncbi.nlm.nih.gov/pmc/articles/ PMC3202683/

Maguire, L. S., O'Sullivan, S. M., Galvin, K., O'Connor, T. P., & O'Brien, N. M. (2004). Fatty acid profile, tocopherol, squalene and phytosterol content of walnuts, almonds, peanuts, hazelnuts and the macadamia nut. International Journal of Food Sciences and Nutrition, 55(3), 171–8.

Mahan, L. K., Escott-Stump, S., & Raymond, J. L. (2012). Krause's Food and the Nutrition Care Process (13th ed.). Elsevier.

Mantzoros, C. S. (2016). Nutrition and Metabolism Underlying Mechanisms and Clinical Consequences. Totowa: Humana Press.

Mason, A., Epel, E., Kristeller, J., Moran, P., Dallman, M., Lustig, R., … Daubenmier, J. Mason, A., Epel, E., Kristeller, J., Moran, P., Dallman, M., Lustig, R., … Daubenmier, J. (2016). Effects of a mindfulness-based intervention on mindful eating, sweets consumption, and fasting glucose levels in obese adults: data from the SHINE randomized controlled trial. Journal of Behavioral Medicine, 39(2), 201–213. https://doi-org.libprox1.slcc.edu/10.1007/s10865-015-9692-8

Meckling, K. A., O'Sullivan, C., & Saari, D. (2004). Comparison of a low-fat diet to a low-carbohydrate diet on weight loss, body composition, and risk factors for diabetes and cardiovascular disease in free-living, overweight men and women. J Clin Endocrinol Metab, 89. https:// www.ncbi.nlm.nih.gov/pubmed/15181047

Melnik, B. C. (2009). Milk--the promoter of chronic Western diseases. Medical Hypotheses, 72(6), 631–9.

Miao, D. (2017). Small Intestinal Bacterial Overgrowth in Modern Bariatric Surgery. Bariatric Times, 14(11), 16–19.

Miller, W. R., & Rollnick, S. (2002). Motivational Interviewing: Preparing people to change (Application). New York: Guilford Press.

Nelson, D. L. (2017). Functional foods: Sources, health effects, and future perspectives. Hauppauge, NY: Nova Science.a

Nielsen, J. V, Jonsson, E., & Nilsson, A. K. (2005). Lasting improvement of hyperglycemia and bodyweight: low- carbohydrate diet in type 2 diabetes. A brief report. Ups J Med Sci, 110.

OSamaha, F. F., Iqbal, N., Seshadri, P., Chicano, K., Daily, D., McGrory, J., … Stern, L. (2003). A low-carbohydrate as compared with a low-fat diet in severe obesity. N Engl J Med, 348. https://www.ncbi.nlm.nih.gov/ pubmed/12761364

Organic Facts. (2017). 9 Wonderful Benefits of Pistachios. Retrieved from https://www.organicfacts.net/health- benefits/seed-and-nut/health-benefits-of-pistachio. html

Orsillo, S. M., Roemer, L., Lerner, J. B., Tull, M. T., Hayes, S. C., Follette, V. M., & Linehan, M. M. (2004). Mindfulness and acceptance: expanding the cognitive-behavioral tradition. (null, Ed.) (Vol. null)

Ozdemir, A., & Buyuktuncer, Z. (2018). Diet, Bariatric Surgery and Gut Microbiota. Istanbul Medical Journal,19(3), 208-213. doi:10.5152/imj.2018.39206

Pagana, K. D., & Pagana, T. J. (2013). Mosby's Manual of Diagnostic and Laboratory Tests (Fifth). St Louis, Missouri: Elsevier - Health Sciences Division.

Patel, S. R., Hayes, A. L., Blackwell, T., Evans, D. S., Ancoli-Israel, S., Wing, Y. K., & Stone, K. L. (2014). The association between sleep patterns and obesity in older adults. International Journal of Obesity, 38(9), 1159–1164. https://www.ncbi.nlm.nih.gov/ pubmed/24458262

Phillips, F. (2011). Dietary issues after bariatric surgery. Independent Nurse, 34–35.

Pinto, G. J., Carvalho, S. A., Palmeira, L., Castilho, P., Duarte, C., Ferreira, C., … Costa, J. (2017). BEfree: A new psychological program for binge eating that integrates psychoeducation, mindfulness, and compassion. Clinical Psychology & Psychotherapy, 24(5), 1090–1098. https://doi-org.libprox1.slcc.edu/10.1002/cpp.2072

Pitchford, P. (2002). Healing With Whole Foods: Asian Traditions and Modern Nutrition (Third). Berkeley, California: North Atlantic Books.

Prietl, B., Treiber, G., Pieber, T. R., & Amrein, K. (2013). Vitamin D and Immune Function. Practical Diabetes,5(7),2502–2521.

Quideau, S. (2009). Chemistry and biology of ellagitannins: An underestimated class of bioactive plant polyphenols. Singapore: World Scientific.

Ralston, S. H., Penman, I. D., Strachan, M. W., Hobson, R. P., Britton, R., & Davidson, L. S. (2018). Davidsons principles and practice of medicine. Edinburgh: Elsevier.

Sanders, T., & Emery, P. (2003). Molecular Basis of Human Nutrition. London: Taylor and Francis.

Sarris, J., & Wardle, J. (2010). Clinical Naturopathy - An Evidence Based Guide to Practice. Churchill Livingstone Elsevier.

Saslow, L. R., Mason, A. E., Kim, S., Goldman, V., Ploutz-Snyder, R., Bayandorian, H., … Moskowitz, J. T. (2017). An Online Intervention Comparing a Very Low-Carbohydrate Ketogenic Diet and Lifestyle Recommendations Versus a Plate Method Diet in Overweight Individuals With Type 2 Diabetes: A Randomized Controlled Trial. Journal of Medical Internet Research, 19(2), 1.

Saslow, L. R., Summers, C., Aikens, J. E., & Unwin, D. J. (2018). Outcomes of a Digitally Delivered Low-Carbohydrate Type 2 Diabetes Self-Management Program: 1-Year Results of a Single-Arm Longitudinal Stud. Journal of Medical Internet Research, 20(8), 2.

Sheard, N. F., Clark, N. G., Brand-Miller, J. C., Franz, M. J., Pi- Sunyer, F. X., Mayer-Davis, E., … Geil, P. (2004). Dietary Carbohydrate (Amount and Type) in the Prevention and Management of Diabetes: A statement by the American Diabetes Association. Diabetes Care, 27(9), 2266–2271.

Sheridan, C. (2016). The mindful nurse: Using the power of mindfulness and compassion to help you thrive in your work. Lexington, KY: Rivertime Press.

Stern, L., Iqbal, N., Seshadri, P., Chicano, K. L., Daily, D. A., McGrory, J., … Samaha, F. F. (2004). The effects of low- carbohydrate versus conventional weight loss diets in severely obese adults: one-year follow-up of a randomized trial. Annals of Internal Medicine, 140.

Sweeney, T. E., & Morton, J. M. (2013). The Human Gut Microbiome. JAMA Surgery, 148(6), 563.

Tamparo, C. D., & Lindh, W. Q. (2012). Therapeutic Communications for Health Care (Fourth). Boston: Cengage Learning.

Teicholz, N. (2014). The big fat surprise. New York, NY: Simon and Schuster.

Templeman, I., Thompson, D., Gonzalez, J., Walhin, J.-P., Reeves, S., Rogers, P. J., Betts, J. A. (2018). Intermittent fasting, energy balance and associated health outcomes in adults: study protocol for a randomised controlled trial. Trials, 19, 1–11.

Turney, J. (2015). I, Superorganism : Learning to Love Your Inner Ecosystem. London: Icon Books Ltd.

Van Wyk, H. (2018). Iron Supplementation. Professional Nursing Today, 22(4), 4–6.

Vattem, D. A., Ghaedian, R., & Shetty, K. (2005). Enhancing health benefits of berries through phenolic antioxidant enrichment: focus on cranberry. Asia Pacific Journal of Clinical Nutrition, 14(2), 120–130.

Vernon, M. C., Mavropoulos, J., Yancy, W. S., & Westman, E. C. (2003). Brief report: clinical experience of a carbohydrate-restricted diet: effect on diabetes mellitus. Meabolic Syndrome and Related Disorders, 1. https://www.ncbi.nlm.nih.gov/pubmed/18370667

Volek, J. S., Sharman, M. J., Gomez, A. L., DiPasquale, C., Roti, M., Pumerantz, A., & Kraemer, W. J. (2004). Comparison of a very low-carbohydrate and low- fat diet on fasting lipids, LDL subclasses, insulin resistance, and postprandial lipemic responses in overweight women. J Am Coll Nutr, 23. https://www. ncbi.nlm.nih.gov/pubmed/15047685\

Volek, J. S., Sharman, M. J., Love, D. M., Avery, N. G., Gomez, A. L., Scheett, T. P., & Kraemer, W. J. (2002). Body composition and hormonal responses to a carbohydrate-restricted diet. Metabolism, 51. https:// www.ncbi.nlm.nih.gov/pubmed/12077732

Webster-Gandy, J., Madden, A., & Holdsworth, M. (2006). Oxford Handbook of Nutrition and Dietetics. Oxford, New York: Oxford University Press, Inc.

Wei, S., Han, R., Shao, J., Wang, S., Huang, M., Wang, & Chen, Y. Intermittent administration of a fasting-mimicking diet intervenes in diabetes progression, restores β cells and reconstructs gut microbiota in mice. Nutrition & Metabolism, Vol 15, Iss 1, Pp 1-12 (2018), (1), 1. https://doi.org/10.1186/s12986-018-0318-3

Sheridan, C. (2016). The mindful nurse: Using the power of mindfulness and compassion to help you thrive in your work. Lexington, KY: Rivertime Press.

Stern, L., Iqbal, N., Seshadri, P., Chicano, K. L., Daily, D. A., McGrory, J., … Samaha, F. F. (2004). The effects of low- carbohydrate versus conventional weight loss diets in severely obese adults: one-year follow-up of a randomized trial. Annals of Internal Medicine, 140.

Sweeney, T. E., & Morton, J. M. (2013). The Human Gut Microbiome. JAMA Surgery, 148(6), 563.

Tamparo, C. D., & Lindh, W. Q. (2012). Therapeutic Communications for Health Care (Fourth). Boston: Cengage Learning.

Teicholz, N. (2014). The big fat surprise. New York, NY: Simon and Schuster.

Templeman, I., Thompson, D., Gonzalez, J., Walhin, J.-P., Reeves, S., Rogers, P. J., Betts, J. A. (2018). Intermittent fasting, energy balance and associated health outcomes in adults: study protocol for a randomised controlled trial. Trials, 19, 1–11.

Turney, J. (2015). I, Superorganism : Learning to Love Your Inner Ecosystem. London: Icon Books Ltd.

Van Wyk, H. (2018). Iron Supplementation. Professional Nursing Today, 22(4), 4–6.

Vattem, D. A., Ghaedian, R., & Shetty, K. (2005). Enhancing health benefits of berries through phenolic antioxidant enrichment: focus on cranberry. Asia Pacific Journal of Clinical Nutrition, 14(2), 120–130.

Vernon, M. C., Mavropoulos, J., Yancy, W. S., & Westman, E. C. (2003). Brief report: clinical experience of a carbohydrate-restricted diet: effect on diabetes mellitus. Meabolic Syndrome and Related Disorders, 1. https://www.ncbi.nlm.nih.gov/pubmed/18370667

Volek, J. S., Sharman, M. J., Gomez, A. L., DiPasquale, C., Roti, M., Pumerantz, A., & Kraemer, W. J. (2004). Comparison of a very low-carbohydrate and low- fat diet on fasting lipids, LDL subclasses, insulin resistance, and postprandial lipemic responses in overweight women. J Am Coll Nutr, 23. https://www. ncbi.nlm.nih.gov/pubmed/15047685\

Volek, J. S., Sharman, M. J., Love, D. M., Avery, N. G., Gomez, A. L., Scheett, T. P., & Kraemer, W. J. (2002). Body composition and hormonal responses to a carbohydrate-restricted diet. Metabolism, 51. https:// www.ncbi.nlm.nih.gov/pubmed/12077732

Webster-Gandy, J., Madden, A., & Holdsworth, M. (2006). Oxford Handbook of Nutrition and Dietetics. Oxford, New York: Oxford University Press, Inc.

Wei, S., Han, R., Shao, J., Wang, S., Huang, M., Wang, & Chen, Y. Intermittent administration of a fasting-mimicking diet intervenes in diabetes progression, restores β cells and reconstructs gut microbiota in mice. Nutrition & Metabolism, Vol 15, Iss 1, Pp 1-12 (2018), (1), 1. https://doi.org/10.1186/s12986-018-0318-3

This is a battle worth fighting.

It is impossible to win the race unless you venture to run, impossible to win the victory unless you dare to battle.
--Richard M. DeVos

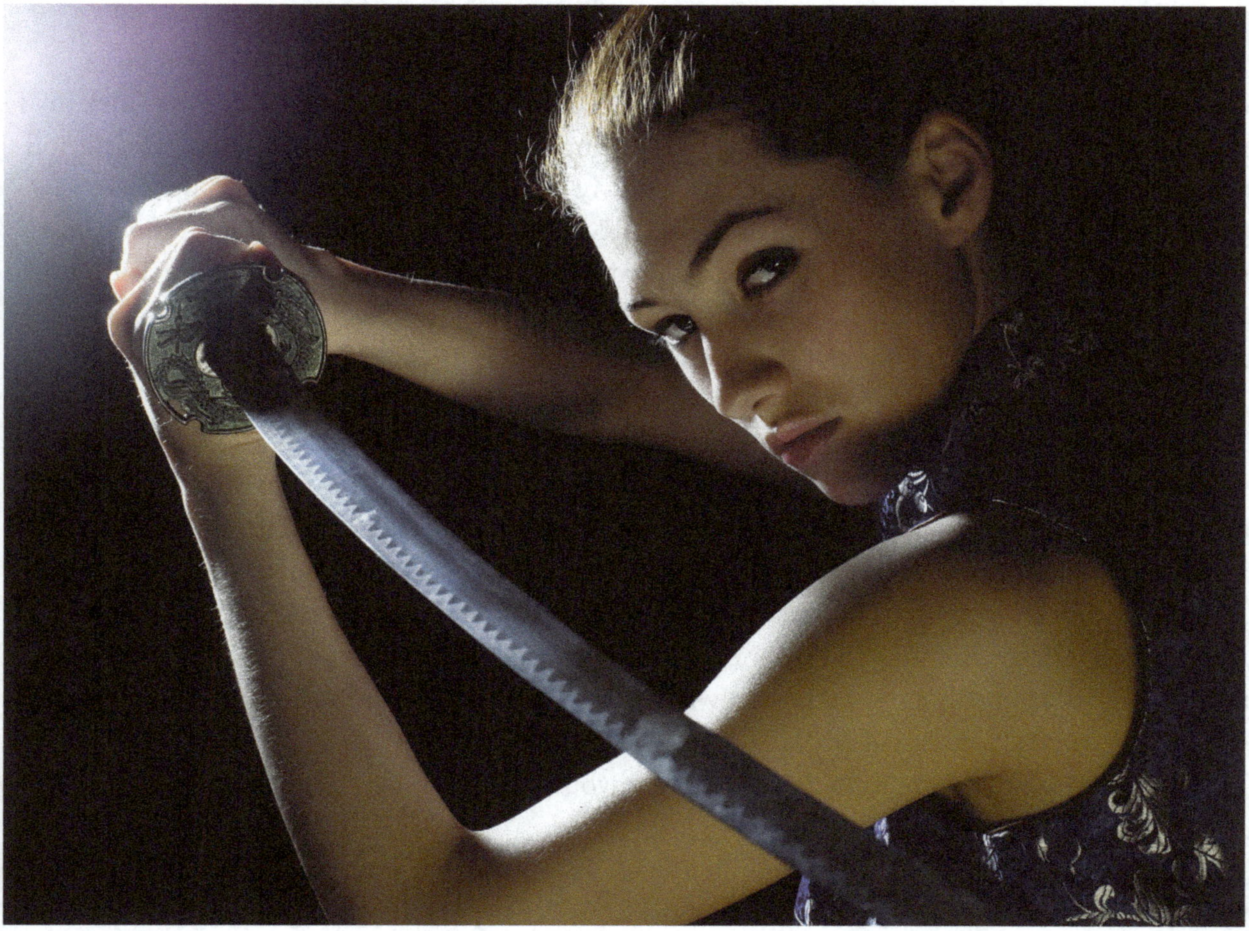

THE BARIKETO STORY

I hold a certificate in Health and Nutrition along with a Master's Degree and a medical research background. When my surgeon expressed WLS hadn't worked well for me, I was crushed. I hadn't lost much weight but figured there was still time for the surgery to "kick in". I had no idea how short the golden honeymoon losing period after weight loss was. The period when the surgery did most of the heavy lifting. My bariatric surgeon told me about Keto but couldn't tell me how to practice it after WLS. Mainstream keto didn't work for me prior to surgery. I didn't have the "willpower". How I hate that word! After surgery the nutrition in mainstream Keto is so far off it can make us sick. So my surgeon tried to get bariatric information on Keto. No one - not me, the surgeon or his staff could find it.

Being a disabled vet, I don't accept defeat easily. I had survived breast cancer after being sent home and told, "There's nothing more we can do for you. Get your affairs in order." Yes, I survived cancer, chemo, radiation & surgery. But I was left a mere shell of myself with no strength. I quickly ballooned to around 350 pounds. I say "around" because I didn't WANT to know how much I weighed. I was ashamed and embarrassed I'd let myself get to that point.. I'd routinely tell the nurse we'd skip the weigh in portion of the doctor's visit and walk straight to the examining room. I was always sick with whatever was "going around". I wasn't willing to go back to that. DAMMIT, I WANTED TO LIVE AGAIN! So I did the only thing I knew to do - I set about creating a program that would work for me.

It took HUNDREDS of hours of research as well as interviewing numerous Bariatric specialists. Members of my November 2016 bariatric surgery support group started to take notice of the sudden shift. One by one I received queries asking what I had changed, and could I help them do it too? The weight loss we achieved was marked enough that others in the group started taking notice.

Some of these amazing women, along with myself, decided to volunteer our time to the bariatric community to help the "slow losers" benefit from our success. That led to the creation of a group called Bariatric Amazons on Keto. We taught the program to over 3K ladies, the majority of whom also lost higher amounts of weight than with WLS alone. The program morphed into this Bariatric Keto program because people couldn't find us under the old name - it was a mouthful!

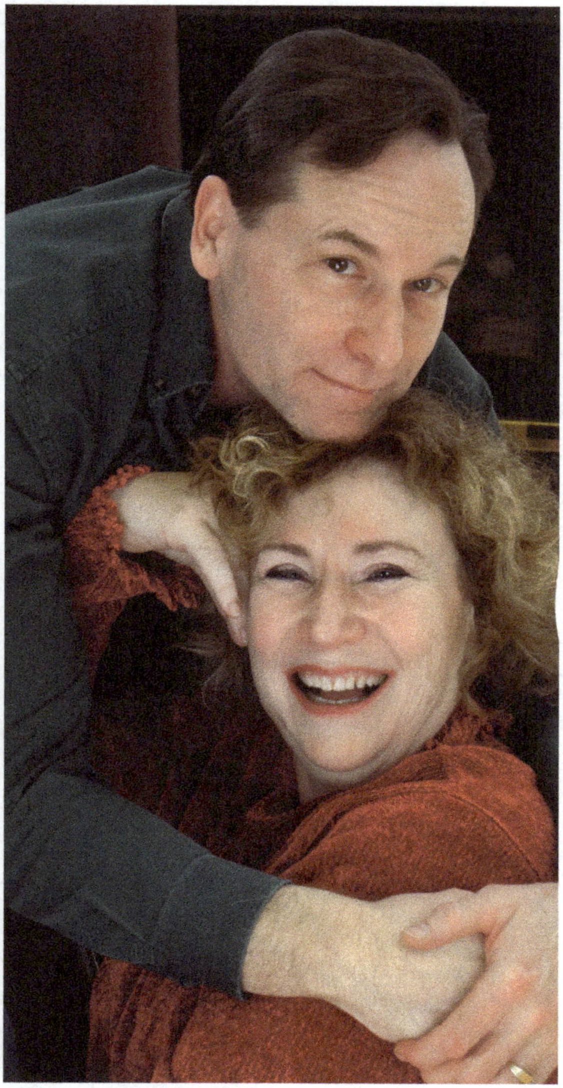

So Bariatric Keto was created totally by accident, born out of a desperate desire to lose weight in a healthy manner. Believe me, if a program had been available I would have followed it rather than taking a year to develop this one! The dozens of moderators you see in our forums are all volunteers who have had WLS and lost successfully with the Bariatric Keto program. They're giving back to the bariatric community by trying to help YOU achieve the same weight loss success. We also have a contributing board of Bariatric Specialists and a Bariatric Dietitian creating menus. Our new menu app is live and can be found in both the Apple & iTunes stores. Like ReStart, the app simply tells you what to eat to help you get to & stay at goal weight. Because that's what we ALL want, and Bariatric Keto makes our clothes fall off.

Author, Mary Beth and Dave, her husband, at their home in Virginia.

CPSIA information can be obtained
at www.ICGtesting.com
Printed in the USA
BVHW010834050721
611060BV00017B/582

9 781087 817255